IRENE TITILOLA OLUMESE

Grace
IN THE
STORMS
A Living Proof

Verbatim

Grace in the Storms - A Living Proof

Copyright © 2017 by Irene Titilola Olumese

Published by **Verbatim Communications Limited**
www.verbatimcomms.com
info@verbatimcomms.com
verbatimcommunications@yahoo.com
+234(0)8133602883, 08180625917

The views expressed in this book are those of the author and do not necessarily represent the views of the publishers.

ISBN: 978-978-52790-7-8

Printed and Bound in Nigeria

"He who is capable of deep and reflective thinking will always be full of gratitude."
(A Yoruba adage).

"When you offer God thanksgiving in the midst of trouble;
that's the purest expression of faith that you can make.
And when you offer Him that thanksgiving you prepare the way in your life, in your heart,
that God may show you His salvation, that God may come to your rescue."
Derek Prince
(www.derekprince.org)

"God never uses anyone greatly until He tests them deeply."
A.W. Tozer

Dedication

To the glory of God, Who called me according to His good purposes to do good works which He prepared ahead of time.

To Peter, Osemudiamen and Ehimenmen;
the three finest men I could ever have asked or prayed for.
You showed me true love and filled my heart with great joy.
May you radiate the light of the glory of God in every sphere of influence God has placed you.
I am blessed to call you my husband and sons.

In honour of my Unknown Benefactor
and organ donors
who give so that others may live.

Acknowledgment

To the Greatest Creative Writer ever known who scripted the story of my life and fitted it into His story I owe all glory and praise for this book. There is not a single portion of this story I would edit or delete if I could. Each chapter is well fitted for His Kingdom agenda.

The writing of this book is a compelling story of life on its own. There were many blocks, hurdles, mountains and valleys along the way. I could not have completed it without the unflinching encouragement of my husband, Peter Olumese, who never stopped reminding me of my uncompleted assignment; "the best cannot be an enemy of good" is still resounding in my ears. Thank you for giving me the permission to bare our lives so publicly, and for bearing with me through the years of developing and writing the book.

To my two sons, Ose and Ehi, whose lives have been exposed in this book, I say; thank you so much for letting me be who you know I needed to be in this book - honest and authentic. This is your story too.

Pastor Patrick Bruce and his wife, Lady Pastor Joy and Sister Cynthia Samuel Olonjuwon, told me at different times almost 15 years ago that I have a story to tell. Thank you for being the three witnesses I needed to confirm the word in my heart. But I didn't know how to tell the story.

Bidemi Mark-Mordi told me that I can write. Though I had for many years been writing the story, an affirmation coming from a seasoned publisher boosted my ego. I am very grateful to Bidemi for the relentless effort she has put into making Grace In The Storm, a dream come true. Heaven knows what you have put in and Heaven will reward you. I am grateful to Ifedolapo Ademosu and the Team at Verbatim Communications who edited the book.

It was at the 2012 Bi-annual Conference of the Geneva Writing Group that I began to hone my skills in writing Creative Non-Fiction. I learnt more at the monthly meeting of the group and many of the Critique sessions. The knowledge and experience shared by the trainers and group members shaped my writing. Thank you for your encouragement.

When it seemed as if the publication of this book would be delayed for much longer, Soji, you stepped in to give a huge push over the looming obstacle. And it was not the first time you and Lara have come to our rescue. You earned yourselves a special place in our family's story as true friends indeed.

I will be eternally grateful to all the doctors, nurses, therapists and aide-soignants who took care of me in more than ten different hospitals in five countries. You have been woven into the tapestry of my life in a special and unforgettable way. Your expertise and skills have been tools in God's hands to keep me here in the land of the living to tell this story.

My heartfelt gratitude and appreciation of the numerous wonderful people, who by the grace of God have been a part of my life in the 50 years of my existence is detailed in the Chapter "Connecting The Dots With Appreciation."

Reviews

The book begins with a beautiful church wedding where Irene and Peter vowed to stay the course of marriage in what is described as "for better for worse, in sickness and in health, for richer and for poorer until death do them part." The story of Irene Titilola spans various countries, from Nigeria to Ghana to Egypt to United States to Geneva. We get a glimpse of a brilliant woman who contributed immensely to UNICEF while raising two young boys and dealing with extremely serious diagnoses. *Grace in The Storms* is a powerful story of a marriage that stood the battering of a debilitating illness and the woman who fought with grace and dignity.

Being diagnosed with a long-term health condition can be frightening and disorienting. Living with a long-term condition can make one particularly vulnerable because of the new layers of stressors. In this book, Irene Olumese has described her journey with considerable details yet what we see throughout the pages is not the illness but the graciousness of the woman who lived each painful experience. Her description of agony and isolation of sickness is tempered with the unconditional commitment of all the individuals and community who were instrumental in each geographic point of her need.

Irene's transparency reminds me of Jesus unveiling his scars to Thomas and invariably to all around him. She writes, "At that point in my life when I was stripped of affluence, spotlight, and audience, there I learnt to trust and obey God." As she trips over the cords of her oxygen tank or watched nurses refusing to come close to her in intensive care or through the incessant bouts of coughing or urinary incontinence, Irene teaches us to dig a little deeper, to hold on for one more moment, and make the effort to do the next best thing. Her tenacity is inspirational! The love story between her and the Lord Jesus Christ is the key to this testimony. Irene permits us entrance into a private relationship with her God who gives her the impetus for life. She writes, "He can restore what has been broken when we hold fast to His word and wait on Him."

In Irene's memoir, we find there is no one too broken for restoration or too lost to be found or too sick to be healed. She writes, "my desire is to fulfil God's purpose and plans for my life, to enter into the fullness of His promises for me."

This is a must read for everyone who is facing challenges in life. In this book, you will find enough grace spilling out of Irene's "Grace in the Storms" to become a living proof.

Dr. Merino - Pastor at Savior's Faith Center. She is a professor and Institutional Vice President and Campus Administrator at Argosy University. Author of several books including Soul Desires, The Perfect Gift of a Mother, Bathtub Therapy, The Keys to Forgiveness and Miracles.

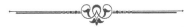

"Grace in the Storms" paints a poignant picture of a lifetime spent trusting in the providence of and depending on God in its *truest* sense. It epitomizes 2 Corinthians 12:9 ("*My grace is sufficient for you, for My strength is made perfect in weakness*" - NKJV) and provides an authentic testament of relying on God even as we pass through the proverbial or literal shadow of death. A must read for all regardless of individual beliefs, but most especially for those struggling with sustaining faith through exceptionally difficult times.

Wale Sobande, PhD - is a husband and father. He resides in Seattle, Washington

Irene's story must be told. This is the amazing true story of an amazing woman that I was privileged to meet and know as a close dear friend.   There are events in the story that I know about because I witnessed them and much more that happened but there is clearly not space enough to include.

Irene is a happy, cheerful, generous, very prayerful, faith filled woman. Her faith and strength in times of adversity is phenomenal. I was the pastor but many times Irene taught us how to pray in a storm, and how to remain optimistic when things looked very dire. She made me appreciate the depth of the statement "Kept by the Power of God," because I saw closely a person who literally lived like that. And she was very personal with her Keeper.

Irene, thank you so much for opening your life in this book to be such a blessing to many more than the few who are privileged to have been able to come close.

Bishop Patrick and Lady Reverend Dr. Joy Bruce - Resident Bishop, True Vine Cathedral, Kumasi, Ghana.

One word sums up Irene's account of her journey so far - MIRACLE!

For the skeptic, this is an eye witness account of instances of divine intervention. For the believer, this is a compendium of testimonies of God's ultimate control, making all things work together for good...

Dr. Olumide Ogundahunsi - Scientist, WHO. Coppet, Switzerland.

If you're at the brink of giving up, this book will give you hope to never ever give up on God and yourself. In the words of Dr. Irene Olumese; "Mountains may shake, earth may quake, and the storms may swirl furiously, cling to hope". Dr Olumese's life is a testimony and challenges me every day. Being a career woman, I could connect with some of her crossroads. Thank you for sharing your story. It has changed my thinking and I know it will change the world.

Mofoluwaso Ilevbare, an Author and a Confidence & Peak Performance Coach lives in Geneva, Switzerland

Foreword

Storms are part of life; they come at varying times often unexpected but occasionally forecasted and they vary in strength and intensity. One unique feature about storms irrespective of its timing and strength is that it will blow away after a while. The critical issue is how strong your anchor is amid the storm? The anchor makes the difference between being blown away with the storm or coming out victorious into clear skies and sunshine on the other side of the storm.

This book is a living testimony of an anchor that not only withstands every possible storm of life, but moulds and refines the vessel with and through the storms. *Grace In The Storms* illustrates the living out of the story of my wife; a story written by God before she was formed in her mothers' womb. I am privileged to have been a part of this story from the very beginning; as a friend, companion, husband and carer among others. It is a story that continues to build and refine my life through each storm and victory.

Grace In The Storms – A Living Proof is not about the strength and toughness of Irene or our family, but rather a testimony of the finished work of Jesus on the cross, when He declared "it is finished," and His resurrection showcased through us in the new life of victory and strength through each storm.

This book takes you through the once-buzzling life of my wife and mother of our two wonderful boys; through a series of medical storms over a period over 21 years that progressed from one degree of severity and intensity to the next until a time when she was completely home-bound and on 24/7 supplemental oxygen and requiring equipment to keep her breathing while asleep; through times of despair and questions as to if God still listens and cares; and through the emotional storms among others. But these situations had the common thread of God providing the needed anchor through the journey even when we almost gave up on hope. When at last, we thought the storm was over with the provision of a second chance at life on this side of eternity through the opportunity of a lung transplant, then arose another major unexpected storm of losing both legs following medical amputation.

Then came the lifting of the clouds and the storm giving rise to the birth of a ministry of inspiring hope and bringing the message of God's amazing grace that is abundantly available to sustain believers through the dark seasons of their lives, and the birth of the Feet of Grace Foundation with the vision that all may walk again.

With ever increasing questions these days as to the purpose of life, should and why Christians suffer, among others, this book cannot be more timely. It testifies of a personal experience of tremendous storms over a 21-year period yet soaring above the storms on eagles' wings proving the faithfulness of God. I recommend this book to everyone. Knowing how to find and hold on to hope amid a storm is critical for survival. This book will surely provide a guide on how to find purpose in your storms through the eyes of our heavenly Father.

It is our prayer that you will find hope and come to the realisation that you are "kept by the Hand of God come what may" as you pass through the stormy and quiet seasons in your life. Always remember that your life is a story pre-written by God before you were formed. Your daily walk in the Lord on this earth is living out that story. His thoughts towards you are for good always to bring you to the expected end, which He had pre-determined.

Never give up on hope; Grace always wins.

Peter Olumese (Husband)
Medical Officer, WHO Headquarters, Geneva, Switzerland

Preface

Storms pay us unexpected visits. Often they come with such stunning ferocity they leave us not only aghast but with a question—where is God in all of this? I have had a sizable share of storms. Sometimes they lined up like incoming airplanes of different sizes flying over my house on their way to Geneva Airport.

Through each storm I came to know the One Who gives peace in the midst of the storm deeper than I knew Him before the storm. I came to know the One Who stills the storms with a command—and that is all it takes.

There was a time that the forceful gale of the whirling storm stole my peace and joy. Soon I found that if firmly rooted on the solid rock, the winds may bellow, waves may rage and I may be swayed but I will never be uprooted from the loving Hands that hold me close to His bosom and His Mighty Hands, which always keep me safe.

My story journals the swiftness with which life can move from calmness to chaos; the transverse from the of fullness of life and strength that once jogged around the perimeter of the University College Hospital in Ibadan, to the extreme that required support and supplemental oxygen to take a few steps. It moved from the freedom of a frequent traveller to the restraining embargo of no travel, from the

> **Through each storm I came to know the One Who gives peace in the midst of the storm deeper than I knew Him before the storm.**

overloaded work schedule to a snow-white agenda, and from the exciting life of outdoor adventures to staring at the trees changing—luscious green to grey dry twigs—through the windows of my bedroom. Through these extremes of life, hope was the fuel that energised me each day and gave me a reason to hold on.

I am thankful to God, that the story did not end with the storms. My story echoes the 126th Psalm of David:
"When the Lord turned again the captivity of Zion, we were like them that dreamt. Then was our mouth filled with laughter, and our tongue with singing: then said they among the heathen, The Lord hath done great things for them.'

"It is a story of amazing recovery, restoration and turnaround for good. God turned it all around and made me a living testimony of His faithfulness and amazing grace."

You will read in this book, testimonies of relentless determination to never give up on hope in the midst of fierce storms. God is not done writing the story of my life. He is still revealing it as it fits His agenda and plan for me. I believe it only ends when Jesus returns or He calls me to glory. So I am holding on; grateful for how far He has brought me and expectant that His hands will continue to hold me up. More than this though is the challenge that you never give up hope no matter what your own peculiar storm may look like.

Table of Contents

Table of Contents

PART ONE

The
STORMS
Begin

The First Decade of Storms

1992 to 2001

No one dreams or envisions a life of crisis, struggles, challenges and storms; certainly not a starry-eyed bride walking down the aisle with her right hand in the crook of her groom's arm and certainly not the groom holding that hand close to his chest. He was charged to defend her with his life if need be. They vowed for better for worse, in sickness and in health, for richer and for poorer until death do them part.

She wore a beaded and sequined bolero over her long white figure-fitted satin dress with sequined appliqués. A cathedral length train trailed behind her. In her left hand was a bouquet of lilac orchids, white roses and green fern. He was in black suit with a silver-grey bow tie and cummerbund. His buttonhole was a miniature of her bouquet. The organ streamed, "Lead us, Heavenly Father, lead us." The couple stole loving glances at one another as family and friends cheered them on with smiles and good wishes.

The bride and groom stepped out of the Chapel into the bright sunny April day, the year was 1992. There was not a single cloud in the blue sky above them. An incredible crowd had gathered around them, even passers-by stopped to watch - truly amazing for a Thursday wedding. They feted over a thousand guests, sang together with a melodious harmony that thrilled guests—at a time when you could not hear the bride's voice save during the exchange of the vows. They danced with friends and families. No one could ask for a more perfect start for a life together.

I was that bride—full of life, energy and passion. My groom and I embarked on our lives' journey together. Unknown to us, a fist-like cloud hung in the horizon. With great hope, big dreams and huge expectations, we taxied the runway and a shaky take off took us to a cruising altitude. We had barely settled down to enjoy the flight, when we hit turbulence—a shocking and unexplainable loss. It was the fourth day of the New Year 1993, when the doctors told me they could not pick foetal heartbeat. I was 32 weeks pregnant. I went through the intense pains of Pitocin-induced labour to deliver a stillbirth. My world spun on its axis as I went back home, empty and empty-handed. But we came out of that storm bonded together and stronger in our resolve to ride upon every storm life brings us. Our loss and grieving together became a turning point in a marriage that was already struggling, and it set us in the right direction towards building a more enriching relationship.

The next storm came under the radar, like a thief in the night. Life was good; lines had begun to fall for us in pleasant places. I got a job that could only be defined as a dream come true as a Nutrition Officer with UNICEF Zonal Office in Ibadan. But I was required to have a medical clearance before my appointment was confirmed. In the interim, I was asked to start working as an in-house consultant filling the post until the required processes were finalised. It was more than a young couple could ask for. Two months later, an incessant and irritating cough that defied treatment made me visit the radiologist for an X-ray. The technician on duty took the first one, reviewed it and called me back to repeat the X-ray. Then he asked me to wait for the Senior Radiologist to review the X-ray. After a long wait, they called me and gave me the report sealed in a white envelope to give to my doctor. "He will explain the results to you," the Radiologist told me.

Although, they did not say a word about their finding, their faces spoke volumes. I quickly succumbed to my curiosity. As soon as I was out of the centre, I opened the envelope and read the report. I did not understand all of it but one word stood out: aneurysm. I had seen that word before and I knew what it meant. I had done an X-ray in 1991 as part of the medical check-up required for a Student Visa when I went to Canada as an Exchange Graduate student. I remembered the doctor told me they noted a shadow in the Chest X-ray, which he said might require further investigation at a later date. I had not given it another thought since I had been cleared to travel. It all came flooding back. I wondered if the shadow was responsible for the latest finding.

Rather than walk straight back home to our apartment, which was by the second gate of the hospital, I took the long route home that evening as my mind went AWOL. I got on the *"Danfo"*, a public bus, from Total Garden to the Hospital Main

Gate and walked the same length back along the circular road. From afar, as I took the last bend, I saw my husband was already back home from work, giving his brown Volkswagen car a shine—his favourite pastime—perhaps to decompress after a stressful day at the Children's Emergency Ward. I paused outside the hibiscus hedge forming the perimeter of the compound, it was in full bloom. I watched my husband for a while over the fuchsia-pink flowers, clutching my hand bag, wondering how I was going to present the report inside the bag to him.

How do you prepare a man for news such as this?

With slow short steps I walked on, he did not notice my approach until I turned into the driveway leading to our block of flats. His hands rested on the brown bonnet of the car glittering under the golden rays of the setting sun as he waited for me. One look at my face, he must have concluded something was not right. For one, I was gone for much longer than normally necessary. In an instant, the doctor's mask dropped and covered his face at the same time he dropped the napkin.
"What is it?"
"Let's go up."

My attempt at remaining calm was fast failing; I needed to get up the flight of staircase to our apartment on the first floor as fast as I could. If you have ever lived with a doctor, you will know they have no room for drama.

"What is it?" He asked the second time, this time with a broach-no-argument tone. I knew him better than to try.

"Not good news." I fingered the white envelope containing the report in my bag and as if time slowed down, my hands still clutching the envelope crawled out of the bag, and handed it to him. Immediately, I turned around and walked up the staircase to our apartment. He paused to read the report. I heard him come up the stairway in quick steps behind me, he entered the apartment with a face that revealed no emotions and said, "Relax, this does not mean anything. They cannot make such a conclusion without further investigation." He flipped the report on the dining table. That was my dear clinician husband comforting me.

We both learned better after several investigations confirmed the presence of a cyst, which at the time was thought to be in my lungs. A bronchoscopy and a life-threatening surgery called thoracotomy followed in June 1993 under difficult circumstances. The surgery had to be postponed thrice within a space of days before it eventually took place. I consistently had a fever the morning of each of the scheduled days for the surgery. The cardio-thoracic surgeons, both Christians, decided to pray about the matter. The next day the surgery was scheduled and they went ahead despite the fever. The surgeons removed what was later found to be a lymphocytic thymoma from between my lungs and heart. I was told it was the size of a fist. The day after the surgery, the Hospital Junior staff went on strike and literally shut down the hospital. We were thankful to God, the surgeons went ahead with the surgery when they did, otherwise it would have been delayed much longer. I made a remarkable recovery and was home five days after. I could no longer stay in the hospital because of the strike. But they continued to monitor me at home. God strategically placed the right people at the right place and at the right time to act on our behalf. This was the first of many God orchestrated events.

We came through that turbulent storm delivered and kept by the mighty hands of God. Although pathologists reported that the cyst was a benign tumour, it created the conditions for another storm; one that lasted a very long time.

#

The Foreboding of a New Storm

Our first son was born in June 1994. His conception and delivery were testimonies of God's remarkable intervention and faithfulness. The umbilical cord had wrapped itself several times around his neck, with every contraction the cord tightened like a noose. It was a close call. So we named him, Osemudiamen, meaning God is standing right by me.

I was back at work four weeks after the delivery. I did not have paid maternity leave because my appointment was yet to be confirmed. I did not get the requisite medical clearance needed in 1993 when I started the job because of my medical condition then. Consequently, I worked as a Temporary staff in a position for which I had been found appointable. The position was re-advertised in the mid of 1994. I re-applied and was interviewed again. After nineteen months of waiting and again by God's divine intervention, I got the medical clearance and my twice-contested appointment as Nutrition Officer at the UNICEF Zonal Office in Ibadan was finally confirmed.

We rejoiced and revelled in the victory and goodness of God in every sphere of our lives. We had a new car, better pay and life was cruising on beautifully at a high altitude...Then another storm hit...

One afternoon in 1995, close to the end of the working day, I had just finished one of those meetings that did not achieve much. I walked along the blue-tiled corridor into my office. It was brightly lit with rays of the setting sun filtering in through the louvered windows from the west side. I closed the door and turned right towards my table. All of a sudden, the room became flooded with light of such blinding intensity that I swiftly swung my hands to cover my eyes. I could have sworn it was an experience similar to that of Saul on his way to Damascus. I blinked and blinked. I could not accommodate the light; it was too intense.

"Where was it coming from?" I wondered as I lowered myself into the visitor's seat in front of me and rested my elbows on the table with one hand holding my head and the other covering my eyes. The fluorescent lamps and sun-rays were indescribably luminous and brilliant. I waited and waited for it go away. I don't know how long I stayed there before it eventually dimmed. The next day, I noticed my eye lids were drooping. I had what is known as "*ptosis*."

I learnt later that my pupils had become fully dilated at that moment, which should only happen in the dark, instead of narrowing as it ought to in the presence of light, therefore giving me the sensation of intense brightness. The sluggish movement of the pupils made it difficult for me to read small print from that point - literally requiring a pair of reading glasses overnight. For a long time, I could not go out during the day without wearing a pair of dark glasses.

It became alarming to watch the expression on the faces of doctors each time they shone their pen touches into my eyes and asked me to follow their fingers, the reaction was always the same. If it was a junior doctor, I could be sure that he or she would call the boss to the scene. The doctors diagnosed what was called, *myasthenic syndrome*. Little did we know that this was the foreboding of a perfect storm, which was already gathering momentum far out in the sea where we had no system for detection.

From then on, I began to suffer from unexplainable allergic reactions. I went from one department in the hospital to the other as we investigated the symptoms that continued to develop.

It was in the midst of all these that I conceived and gave birth to our second son in August 1997. We named him, Ehimenmen, meaning "God is good indeed." The name testifies of God's goodness in keeping me through the difficult season. The fully paid four-month long maternity leave provided me with much needed rest. The strain of the cough which had remained unabated was taking its toll on me, both physically and emotionally.

#

The Perfect Storm

High flying with high profile jobs and the emerging comfort of accomplishment in different spheres of our lives, suffice to say my husband and I were unprepared when the next storm struck. This time it was more ferocious than before. It churned and threatened. It whirled and raged. Nothing was left untouched. We began to ask questions as we noted that the storms seemed to come with startling cyclical regularity - each one more devastating than before. Like storm watchers, we examined the pattern of the storms closely and remembered that the House Officer who took my medical history during a major hospitalisation in 1986 unwittingly hinted of this pattern. We thought we had dealt with the issue since that first indication, but we came to an unnerving and unavoidable conclusion: we were wrestling not against flesh and blood but against spiritual wickedness in heavenly places. The networking of this spiritual wickedness was uncanny.

July 1998

The year was 1998. I was under pressure to finish my long-drawn out doctorate programme. Working full time as a Nutrition Specialist with 40% travel, and nursing my six-month old second son meant that I had to burn my candles at both ends to accommodate the demands of writing my thesis. I practically worked round the clock for six months to prepare my thesis for defence, scheduled for the 31st of July, 1998.

A spiritual battle was unleashed behind the scenes on the day of the defence. I experienced the wickedness of men in their unrelenting effort to frustrate a fellow human being with such great evil intent and in a personal way too, as never before. The opposition was intense. The people I had once held in high esteem were intent on ensuring that the examination did not take place as scheduled. Important documents suddenly disappeared from my academic file to present a situation that I did not complete the requirement for the examination. They demanded a rescheduling of the examination. The external examiner who came from another university was already seated. The implication of rescheduling the examination was that I would no longer qualify for the award of the degree even after a successful defence because I would have exceeded the number of semesters allowed by the University's regulation for the completion of a doctorate programme.

Once again, God intervened and raised up a 'Gamaliel' to speak on my behalf. It was only by this divine intervention that I was allowed to defend my doctorate thesis on the same day seven hours after the scheduled time. I emerged on the other side after several hours of grilling that ran into the night, recommended to be awarded the degree: Doctor of Philosophy in Nutrition Sciences. A journey of almost ten years successfully completed. But that was not the end of the battle.

The relentless effort to frustrate my work did not end on that day. In the coming months, this same group of persons continued to stand against my interests and made every possible attempt to manipulate the system in order to prevent my book from being approved by the Postgraduate Committee of my Faculty and to ensure that I was not enlisted for the Convocation. God, in His infinite mercies stretched a finger of resistance against them and exposed their evil machinations at the highest authority. It took an executive order from the Provost of the College of Medicine to ensure that my book was approved and I was enlisted for the convocation scheduled for November of the same year.

While the warfare was in full force to stall my academic progress, my health came under attack again. The gale was fierce. It swept me off balance and would have swept me away but for the mighty hands of God that anchored me firm to the rock. We certainly did not see this coming.

The Meltdown

I was in the middle of a presentation at a training workshop organised by the Country Office when I noticed that I was slurring and it felt as if the muscles in my nasal tract and throat were melting. I paused, stopped talking, swallowed hard and coughed several times in the bid to create space for breathing. I summarised and concluded the presentation in a slow and low tone voice but as quickly as I could muster the strength. I was confused at what was happening to me and yet did not want to draw any attention to myself. I escaped to the bathroom immediately afterward.

Over the next few days, I noticed a worrisome and remarkable weakness in the muscles in my face and upper body. The coughing at this time had worsened, making breathing very difficult. From thence on, I literally spiralled downhill. The weakness in my upper muscles made it difficult for me to even comb my hair. I could not hold my hands up. I had to put my head on my lap to comb and style my hair every morning. The incessant coughing was choking life out of me.

One morning soon after I returned back home from the training workshop, I was bathing my second son when my arms went limp. The baby slipped from my hands into the bath tub. Thankfully, it was a plastic tub and the water was shallow. Shaken, I called out to my brother-in-law living with me at the time to finish bathing the boy and went back into my room.

"What's going on?" my heart cried out to the Lord.

"How was I going to get through the day in this state of sheer debilitation?" I wondered.

I had scheduled a meeting with Breastfeeding Assessors coming from eight states of the South-West Zone. I needed to be in the office for this exercise to go on as scheduled. I called for help to get to the office. Driving myself was not an option, my pupils were dilated again and I was having difficulties accommodating the bright afternoon sunlight on top of the weakness and the aggravating cough. With my hands partly supporting my head and partly blocking off the light, and with all the strength I could muster, I attended to the Assessors and got them on their way.

Against the advice of my colleagues at work, I went back home instead of heading straight to the hospital. But my sister-in-law came home to stay with me. It was the mighty hands of God that kept me through that night when I got down to the valley of the shadow of death. My husband was away from home on an official assignment in Kenya. My sister-in-law sat on the floor with me through the night because I could not lay down on the bed without gasping for breath. It was a very long night. I coughed relentlessly. My chest was burning as if on fire. It was difficult to breathe. She and her brother called in our family friend, Prof. JO, who is a doctor as soon as the day broke. He came with my Chest Physician, Dr. OI. One look at me and Dr. OI told me we needed to get to the hospital immediately.

The first night in the hospital was a nightmare, I had been on oxygen supplementation all day but it was not humidified and I began to have a massive headache so painful that I could not sleep that night. I was greatly distressed. By the following day, I found myself in the Intensive Care Unit of the University College Hospital in a battle for my life. A condition diagnosed as *Myasthenia Gravis,* a degenerative disease of the neuromuscular junction, coupled with oxygen insufficiency as a result of an inconclusive respiratory disease was threatening my life.

Beyond the physical manifestations we were seeing, the battle was also intense in the spiritual realm. Strange events occurred there in the intensive care unit. One night, a matron from another ward came into the ICU. She stood at the door and shouted,

"Irene Olumese, Bed 6!" I was startled. Her voice reverberated across the room.

She turned around and walked out of the Unit. Stunned at the strange behaviour of a senior nurse, one of the ICU nurses ran after her but she came back looking perplexed. I lay on my bed in the white-walled ward wondering what that was about. The storm took a new dimension that night. I felt I was in the middle of a tug-of-war between two forces - being pulled forcefully in opposite directions.

At some point, I heard a choir singing. I was unsure where the melodious song was coming from. I thought they were angels singing from the direction behind my bed.

As the enemy waged war in the heavenly places, friends and families went on their knees in prayers. God raised up a standard against the enemy and delivered me by His mighty hands. I came out of that experience with Psalm 124 ringing in my head - "If it were not for the Lord on my side, when the enemy rose up against me, then they would have swallowed me up quick."

I was eventually discharged to go home and given a medication to control the *Myasthenia Gravis;* but still no solution was found for the cough except to palliate it with several sessions of inhalation each day.

Kept By the Power of Jesus

Back at home, I continued to struggle with the coughing. It was rib-cracking and painful. My throat and chest felt like they were on fire after each severe bout of coughing. I spent hours each day doing steam inhalation with menthol. The menthol stung my eyes and added to the distress.

The side effects of the medications taken to control the *Myasthenia Gravis* made me to start hallucinating. Every morning, I would tell my husband that I did not sleep through the night, yet I would recount with vivid clarity the weird dreams and visions I saw throughout the night. It was as if I was in a state of limbo of some sort, in between a conscious and subconscious state where I did not have the rest of proper sleep and yet was not fully awake. Most of the dreams and visions were frightening. It was evident that we were in spiritual warfare. My husband began to play Toun Soetan's gospel cassette throughout the night. I found myself waking up during the night to hear "Kept by the power of Jesus. Kept by the power of God, day by day and come what may. I am kept by the hands of God." This line of the lyrics streamed into my sub-consciousness and became a constant reminder that I am kept by God's mighty hands as the enemy unleashed his relentless attack on me. It was at this time that I started having difficulties to control my bladder. The more I coughed, the more difficult it became for me to hold back the leaks. The cough still remained relentless despite the aggressive treatment.

This was the state of my health when I went for the Convocation Ceremony to receive my doctorate degree on November 13th, 1998 at the University of Ibadan. Dressed in a lime green pantsuit, I walked up the incline from the car park

> Again, I had to choose whose report I was going to believe. I rejected the doctors' prognosis and made up my mind to live my life to the fullest as God gives me the grace.

along the road in front of the Bellamy Hall to the Trenchard Hall. I held my handbag and a plastic bag to hold the used tissue paper as I continued to produce large quantities of secretions from my chest. My husband carried my red gown, blue cap and lime-green hood in one hand, and held me to support me as we walked. It felt as if with every step we look the road was rising up to meet me, and the road suddenly became steeper. I was out of breath, panting and coughing by the time we got to the place where we were expected to line up for the procession. A couple of friends who saw us coming quickly found a place for me to sit down while my husband solicited their help to support me as we began the procession into the Hall.

All hell broke loose on that day, when a student's protest broke out against the presence of one of the dignitaries invited for the convocation. The police in response threw canisters of tear gas to disperse the protesting students. The Convocation ceremony came to an abrupt halt as the fumes from a burning car began to fill the hall. A stampede erupted as Graduands and their guests rushed out of Trenchard Hall. Despite the rush to leave the hall, no one pushed me off where I was seated. It was as if I was surrounded by an invisible protective shield from the crowd. I could not move from my seat without assistance. I was rooted to that spot watching the fumes coming through the top windows in front of the hall. I remembered pleading with God that the fumes must not get to where I sat immobile, knowing fully well the implication for my already compromised respiratory system.

God kept guard over my life and miraculously delivered me from every fiery arrow shot at me. My husband eventually found his way into the hall to find me on my seat waiting for help. We got out of the hall after the crowd had left. Incredibly, the security situation was brought under control after a couple of hours and the Convocation ceremony resumed. But it was concluded without the usual pomp. That did not matter. What mattered the most to me was that despite all the arsenal the enemy unleashed from all directions to prevent me from getting this degree, God intervened to confound his plots and to bring me victory. In all the pandemonium, I did not remember to take any photograph. By the time we got back home, I had to rest. I could not attend to all the guests who came to celebrate with us. I learnt much later that many of our guests were puzzled and left wondering what was going on with us.

One question kept gnawing at my heart for many years later; "What was so critical about this academic achievement that the host of hell unleashed such fury to prevent it?"

I wondered why all these events were happening. I wondered about the purpose of it. One thing I knew for sure was that God was aware of all the networks of wickedness arrayed against me and He was more than able to keep me through it all. I still don't have an answer to this question but I am persuaded that all these are not chance events; they are tiny pieces of a large puzzle God is building of my life. The picture will become clearer at God's appointed time.

By the end of 1998, I had a fairly good idea of what I was battling against. Five years already into the struggle with my health, I knew the battle line had been drawn. But still I went on to get a second opinion from doctors in USA. The report they gave me was unnerving as it confirmed the diagnosis made by my doctors in Nigeria. The outlook was that as the degenerative neurological disease progressed, it would become more difficult for me to carry out my daily activities without support, and I may eventually require a wheelchair to move around, and assistance to do basic things. This situation was further complicated by the respiratory disease, which at this time was diagnosed as *Bronchiectasis*. We did not have any answers as to what had triggered the condition.

Again, I had to choose whose report I was going to believe. I rejected the doctors' prognosis and made up my mind to live my life to the fullest as God gives me the grace. Armed with a medication that I was required to take 3-4 times a day to slow down the progression of the disease, I returned to Nigeria in February 1999.

#

Finding Balance in Conflicting Roles:

A few months after I returned home, my office was relocated from Ibadan to Ikoyi in Lagos. And that began another chapter of my story - a story of dealing with a debilitating disease while working under difficult circumstances. The next two years were challenging for me as a professional seeking to make my mark in my chosen field, as a defender of the rights of the staff members in the organisation, as a wife and mother commuting between two cities 140 kilometres apart, and then as a manager of a sub-office with twenty-five staff members. All of these, in the presence of the relentless attack on my health and uncertain career growth.

The new role required me to live in Lagos and meant I had to commute a longer distance from home to work every day in heavy traffic and breathing in air polluted by fumes. I did not have my car with me at the initial period. I took a taxi to and from work; I had to walk a significant distance from my brother's in Anthony Village, and cross a major highway in

> **My husband picked up the broken pieces, and put it all together again before sending me back to prepare the office for my new boss.**

order to get the taxi to go to work. The stress was complicating my health situation. I decided to hire a taxi at a huge cost that would take me right from the doorstep of the house to work. After a few months of this arrangement, I developed a severe allergic reaction. I knew it was as a result of the polluted air.

Several nights, I was awoken by severe itchy weals on my body. Sometimes, I woke up to find my lips and face swollen. It got to the point that I needed to learn to administer steroid injections by myself whenever these reactions flared up.

It was in the midst of these struggles that a very dear friend and colleague, Sweet Giwa-Osagie, offered to accommodate me in her home. She lived just about 15 minutes' drive to my office. Though, the frequency of the allergic reactions reduced during this time, I began to have severe bone pain crisis similar to that experienced by patients suffering from sickle cell anaemia. My blood type is AS but under extreme stress, I tend to sickle more and experience bone pain. The pain got worse and became more frequently. The stress of living in Lagos, the work environment and commuting weekly between Lagos and my home in Ibadan took a huge toll on my health. I began to take a heavy painkiller to control the bone pain.

That was when I decided to find an accommodation in Ikoyi close enough to the office. Unfortunately, by this time also, I had developed a stress-induced abdominal ulcer. I was not eating well and regularly. I was taking a lot of different medications that were eroding the lining of the wall of my stomach. It was in Lagos I knew what excruciating pain truly meant. Between the bone pain and the pain from the ulcer, on several occasions I found myself rolling on the floor in pain. There was a day, the pain started in the night, but I had a crucial meeting in the morning and could not stay back at home. I went to the meeting and was in great pain and distress throughout the meeting. I was eager for the meeting to be over and for the partners to leave my office. I was the Officer-in-charge of the Zonal Office at this time. I still don't know how I managed to keep a straight face and sit still throughout the meeting. When the partners left my office, I fell on my knees by the sofa, and began to weep and groan in pain. That was where my secretary found me about an hour later. The pain washed over me in wave after wave relentlessly. Nothing I took or did helped. I knew I had to get back to Ibadan to see my doctor. I called my driver in and we began the 161km drive from my office to my home.

The storm passed and I was back in the office the following week, after spending a couple of nights in the hospital to investigate and deal with the pain. God gave me the grace to keep up with my work in the midst of these health challenges. Grace was the fuel that kept me going. The last thing I wanted was for the quality of my work to fall as a result of my health. I clung to God for leading, guidance, direction, and wisdom each day in order for me to navigate the stormy waters of my multiple workloads in the office as both the Nutrition Specialist and the Officer-in-charge managing the day-to-day administration of the office.

In Search of Career Growth

At some point, I applied for the post of the Head of the sub-office, a post I was already occupying as the Officer-In-Charge. The selection process was intense and rigorous with a full day of written test. The written test was so intense that several applicants both internal and external walked out of the room in frustration. I was short-listed for an interview following the test. The interview was one of the most challenging I have ever attended in my life. The hostility exuding from one of the members of the interview panel was palpable. I knew her very well and I will refer to her as the Madame. We had disagreed on many issues that bordered on the high premium I felt the organization should place on its human resources. As the Chairperson of the Staff Association, I had to defend many staff related issues in the face of the management approach she pushed. We also disagreed on her approach to the management of the Nutrition component of our programming work. I knew she did not like my guts but I did not appreciate the depth of her dislike of me until that day. She brought out all these issues during the interview to present a case that I was too staff-orientated and too mono-directional in my qualifications as a science specialist to be a suitable candidate for the management position. The venom the Madame spewed from across the room stung me beyond words. I was there for hours without being offered a glass of water to the extent that my mouth was so dry, my tongue clung to the roof of my mouth that I had to intermittently pause to salivate.

At the end of the interview, which was the longest of all the interview sessions conducted that day, I felt battle-worn; physically, emotionally and spiritually exhausted. It was one of the most stressful days of my life. I was not in the least surprised when I got the hint that the Madame had strongly opposed my promotion and appointment as the substantive Head of the zonal office. But I was most unprepared to learn a few weeks later, that an external candidate had been appointed to the post.

> **I learnt the lesson again that the anger of man does not produce the righteousness God desires.**

I went back home to my husband and children feeling cheated out of a unique and very rare opportunity for career growth within the organization. My self-esteem was shattered to smithereens. My husband picked up the broken pieces, and put it all together again before sending me back to prepare the office for my new boss. I needed a super-abundant supply of grace to keep my head and spirit high in the weeks that followed. The strain of managing the office under this additional stress as well as managing full time my primary responsibility as the Nutrition Officer continued to batter my health.

It was indeed the grace of God that kept me from being bitter against the Madame, who was my superior officer. It was with grace that I prepared the office and handed over its management to the new boss. But guess what? Before the scheduled arrival, I went on an emotional shopping spree. I bought myself the most expensive pant suit I have ever owned. It was an Italian silver-grey silk suit. I wore the suit and an immaculate white blouse with grace on the day of arrival of my new boss. The silver stripes made me feel very tall and professional. Believe me, I simply needed the outfit to boost my self-esteem. I went first to the Country Office to meet with my new boss in a meeting with the Madame who was the supervising officer for the post. I was not going to give the Madame any reason to gloat or to think she got under my skin. I was determined to be very professional in my appearance and in all my dealings with her and the new Head of Office. So I worked extremely hard and gave every due attention to detail as I prepared and presented the report of the status of programme implementation in the zone and my handing over notes.

It was grace that kept me working in office under the new boss with an uplifted face when everyone else expected me to be downcast in the midst of this challenging situation, which included showing my boss the ropes about our programming work in the Zone. That grace earned me the respect of my colleagues and the staff members.

At A Crossroad

I was back in the USA in December 2000 for a medical check-up. My friends and family there pleaded with me to relocate to the US. They felt that I would have access to better medical services to manage the many ailments I faced. I did not get a go-ahead in my heart about this and neither did my husband. And I had no plans of relocating to the US without my husband and children. At the same time, the path for an upward career growth in my organization was very dim. I was tired of the system. I was tired of incessant opposition. Yet, I knew I could not just stay back in the US.

I was at this cross-road of decision-making on a snowy morning in January 2001. I had just helped my hostess to tidy up the house while they attended to their new-born babies in the hospital. I stood by the window of their bedroom; it was pristine white outside, sun beams made the snow glitter like diamonds.

My heart swelled up within me, "Lord, I need to hear a word from you" I cried out.

With much longing to know what God wanted me do, I fell on the floor, laid prostrate on the soft cream carpet and poured out my heart out to God. I asked Him to open a door for my husband to get a post in an international organization. I wanted global recognition for my husband and his work. I told the Lord that I was ready to trade the possibility of my getting an international post in my organization for my husband to get one. Unknown to me, my husband was also praying and asking God to give me an opportunity for an international appointment in return for work I had put into the organization. I found out about his prayers later.

God, who works in ways beyond our imaginations to perform His wonders in our lives, chose to answer both our prayers. He opened the door for my husband to get what began as a short term appointment for six weeks at the WHO headquarters in Geneva. And against all the odds, I got an international appointment as a Nutrition Specialist in the UNICEF office in Ghana. Incredibly, the Madame gave me such a glowing recommendation that I was convinced she could not have written it herself. Someone must have drafted it for her and compelled her to send it or her desire to get me out of the office was so great that she did not mind writing such a recommendation. Either way, I knew it was by God's intervention because all I had afterward was a call from the Accra office offering me the post on the strength of the recommendations. By April 2001, I was on my way to Tamale in the Northern Region of Ghana to commence my assignment and the next chapter of my story, unaware of when the next storm would touch down.

Earlier in 1999, I was at a Health and Nutrition meeting convened by the then Head of the Section, the Madame. They had moved the motion to merge the Nutrition programme with the Health programme, which I strongly objected to because under the Health Section, Nutrition would be restricted to a prescriptive component. Nutrition as a programme has a huge social component and relates with several other professionals in other sectors beyond the Health Sector. At this meeting, the first one for the two merged sections, the Head of the Section proposed to limit the full-fledged Nutrition Programme to just the Micronutrient project and moved to scrap the remaining projects under the Nutrition programme. As if this was not bad enough, she proposed to reclassify the post of the Nutrition Officers to a lower level. Needless to say, I was livid. I watched the years of labour building the Nutrition programme in the country evaporate like a vapour and disappear into thin air.

In anger; yes I do get very angry and can be hot-tempered but God's grace helps me to keep it under check, I packed my stuff, carried my bag and stomped out of the meeting room. I was not listening to the voice of the Holy Spirit to manage my emotions. I was very upset and felt helpless and unable to prevent this demolition plan. But alas, in my very high heeled black court shoe, I missed the step and rolled all the way down the staircase. The pain was excruciating; I had sprained my ankle. But that was not the worst of the pain. More painful was having the same people I was debating with and angry with standing at the top of the stairway commiserating with me. That was very painful. I learnt the lesson again that the anger of man does not produce the righteousness God desires. I spent the next day in bed and had to do an X-ray to exclude the possibility of a fracture in my ankle. I limped with my ankle immobilized for the duration of the meeting. As you can imagine, I remained quiet throughout. I had lost this particular battle but I made it quite clear that it was a bad decision. Of course, this did not put me in the good books of the Madame.

Unbeknown to us, I had sustained an internal injury in my hips. I apparently hit the head of my femoral bone against the socket when I had the fall. It was about a year later that I began to have severe pains in my hip especially in the night when I lay on that side of my hips and during the day when I wore very high shoes. It was bad enough for me to have to stop wearing high-heeled shoes—humph! I also walked like a duck in flat shoes. The pain eventually got out of hand and I had to see an orthopaedic surgeon. That was when we discovered that I had an inflammation on the head of the femoral bone. He asked me if I had a fall in the past. I remembered my inglorious fall in anger the year before. He prescribed some anti-inflammatory drugs, which he said would only provide a short-term respite from the pain. He strongly suggested that I consider a surgical intervention that would leave me immobilized for about six months. He was willing to make the arrangements for me to have the surgery in the UK.

I was in shock as we left the Surgeon's office. That spur of uncontrolled anger was costing me more than I could have imagined. This was coming after I had already committed to taking the position in Ghana. Six months of being immobilized was not an option to consider. I cried to the Lord to heal me and blot out the pain. It was with a limp on low-heeled pumps that I headed to Ghana. I will share the testimony of God's miraculous intervention later in this book.

PART TWO

Still At It
The Second Decade of

STORMS

(2001 to 2012)

A New Beginning in an Unknown Place

"I will go ahead of you, and make the crooked places straight:" (Isaiah 45:2). God promised in Isaiah 42:16 that He will take the hand of those who don't know the way, who can't see where they're going. He promised to be their personal guide, directing them through unknown country. "I will be right there to show them what roads to take, make sure they don't fall into the ditch. These are the things I am doing for them, sticking with them, not leaving them for a minute" (The Message paraphrased).

This was indeed the testimony of my relocation to and sojourn in Ghana with my two sons. During my first trip I found out that the office where I was to be based was not as close to Accra as I had earlier thought. It was, in fact, almost eleven hours by road, located in a town called Tamale in the Northern Region of Ghana. My first flight was in an F-27 Fokker plane managed by Sobel Air with a capacity for sixteen passengers; it was the smallest plane I had ever been on. I had a prayer in my mouth throughout the journey.

The single lane coal-tarred narrow road from the airport into Tamale was bordered mostly by fields of guinea corn and millet, but soon small white bungalows appeared sparsely scattered along the way with twig fences forming the outer perimeter of the compounds. More buildings appeared as we drew closer to the town. The air was very hot and dry. And this was just the beginning of the dry season.

The Lord went ahead of us to prepare the place for us. He divinely connected us with the Pastor of the Lighthouse Church International. The family of three boys became buddies for our boys in a strange land. The church became our home church and we were surrounded by people who received us with warmth and kindness. The Bruce family became a conduit of God's blessings to us, during the season of calmness, and a great support when storms broke loose again.

I found a house with a very big compound to rent. It shared a fence with my office. The dilapidated three-bedroom bungalow was renovated and the compound cleared of the overgrown trees. It was painted white. Fully air-conditioned with dark green curtains made from Nigerian tie and dye fabric, the house was kept cool and shielded from the dry desert heat. My boys had a large enclosed ground to play and ride their bicycles in safety, while I worked long hours away from home.

My work in Ghana involved frequent traveling within the Northern Region, between Tamale and Accra where the country office was based, and outside the country. With my husband now based in Geneva at this time, we also had to oscillate between Geneva, Ghana and Nigeria. We were kept by the mighty hands of God during all these journeys. I had the challenge of how to ensure my children were properly cared for during my frequent absences. God, in His faithfulness raised up family members and friends who took turns to come to Ghana to take care of the boys in addition to the support provided by my housekeeper and nanny there. This gave me the opportunity to do my work with my mind at rest.

During my stay in Ghana, the cough remained relentless in its pursuit, draining me of energy and compounded my already stressful work life. It got to a stage that I became heavily dependent on *Benylin* with Codeine to suppress the cough especially during the many presentations I had to give and many meetings I had to attend. Staying wide awake and vibrant with the codeine in my blood stream posed a challenge. I had stopped drinking coffee since my late teenage years when I started having rapid heart rates after taking coffee. So I drank several cups of tea and nibbled on snacks to keep me alert. This resulted in rapid weight gain. Suppressing the cough also meant that I was not effectively evacuating the secretions in my chest. The accumulation of these secretions resulted in chronic chest infection requiring frequent antibiotic treatments.

During my second year in Ghana, my husband applied for a higher position in WHO which would ensure that he had a longer term contract with the organization and better benefits both for himself and the family. We learnt that he performed very well during the interview but we had to wait patiently for the appointment to be announced. We knew God was working behind the scenes on our behalf, using his team leader. We knew it was necessary to ensure that the environment where he would be working would be conducive for him after the announcement was made. But we did not know it would take as long as it did.

Caught in a Turbulence

One bright sunny day early in 2003, I set out on a trip to Accra on my way to Lagos to attend to family matters in Ibadan. It was by air on the usual F-27 plane. We soon hit a turbulent storm as we approached the Eastern Region of Ghana. The plane became like a ribbon tossed up and down in a whirlwind as we flew over the densely-forested mountainous range. The pilot's cabin door flew open as the plane vibrated with vigour, and I saw heavy drops of sweat dripping down the face of the pilot on the right seat from my front row seat on the left side of the plane. It might as well have been raining in the cabin. As the winds lifted the plane up to the heavens and pushed it down again into the valley, my heart dropped to the pit of my tummy and the passengers screamed. The hostess sitting on the other side of the aisle was visibly shaking. She held her head over her knees in a braced position. I knew we were in a grave situation. The plane spun like a top and reeled like a drunkard with the force of the turbulent winds. Someone once told me that it is almost impossible to find planes that went down over the mountain range in the past. I looked out of the window into the heavy dark clouds and cried out to the Lord in my heart. "I will not die in this storm," I declared and continued to pray in the spirit.

God heard my cry and got us out of that desperate situation just in the nick of time. He quieted the storm and delivered us from the horror of a plane crash. Thrown off course, it took twice as long as the normal travel time but the Lord brought us safely back on course to the airport at Accra. As soon as we disembarked from the plane, nearly all the passengers fell to their knees right there on the tarmac to give thanks to God. It was when I switched on my phone that I saw several missed calls from my husband. I called him back immediately to tell him of the wonderful deliverance God wrought on my behalf and relieve his apparent anxiety. My joy was doubled as he delivered the wonderful news to me - his appointment as a P5 Medical Officer with WHO was announced shortly after my flight took off from Tamale.

It was with great joy that I ran to the check-in counter for my onward flight to Lagos, praising God all the way. While on board the plane praising God, the magnitude of what God had done hit me like a thunderbolt and jolted me upright in my seat. If the plane had crashed as it could most likely have, had the good Lord not intervened on our behalf, my husband's joy would have been cut short by the news of the crash and the ensuing sorrow. It took my praise to another level. But it soon appeared I was not out of the woods yet for that day. Just as the plane approached the airport in Lagos, it suddenly became pitch dark on the ground - electricity had gone off. Praise be to God; the pilot was able to land the plane safely without a hitch. It was with exhilarating joy that I planted my feet on a firm ground as we disembarked and I exited from the plane. I could not but marvel at the faithfulness of God and be grateful for His marvellous love to us. All I wanted to do was to lift up a high praise to Him.

#

Kept By The Hands of God

The cough took a turn for the worse in April 2003, right in the middle of the preparation for an international workshop I was organizing to review the status of the operational research ongoing in some of the focus communities I was responsible for. I had been coughing much more than before for three weeks nonstop. It became almost impossible to get a good night sleep because of the intensity of the cough. I started having several episodes of respiratory difficulties during the day and night. I had to take a road trip to Accra at this time to attend several meetings at the Country Office and to finalise some arrangements for the workshop at the Country Office. I also wanted to see the doctor at the UN Clinic as I was very uncomfortable with the cough and the pain in my chest.

The doctor initiated a course of oral antibiotic treatment based on the volume and colour of the expectoration, and asked me to come see him the following week for further investigations. To quieten the cough and get some relief especially during the day while at meetings, I went back to using *Benylin* with codeine. I had to use this medication several times one night to get some respite from the cough and so that I could finalise my presentation for the meeting in the morning. I was in pain and restless. I could not find any position comfortable enough to do my work or to sleep for that matter. I eventually finished the presentation at almost 4:00am. I knew I must sleep if I was to cope with the heavy schedule ahead of me that day.

The rib-cracking cough refused me any rest. It was simply by the sheer grace of God that I got through my presentations and meetings that day. It was in this condition that I headed back to Tamale a couple of days later. I could not wait in Accra until the following week to go back and see the doctor. I had barely a week to the International Conference and I wanted to be with my children. The 11-hour road trip back to Tamale seemed extremely long and tortuous. I was restless as I struggled to breath. I arrived in Tamale exhausted.

The next few days were intense, while my brain was in overdrive preparing for the international meeting; the situation with my health took a turn for the worse. It was very difficult to breathe especially when lying down and it felt like a heavy stone weighed down on my chest whenever I lay down. I had to prop up on the pillows and sat up through the night to get some rest. I was in distress the following day. It was Sunday, getting out of bed was not an option. I was too ill to go to Church so I sent a message to Pastors Patrick and Joy. They came over to the house after the service. We talked about what was going on. They encouraged me and prayed with me. It felt like having a family with me.

By the following morning, the situation turned grave as I struggled to breathe. I knew this had gone beyond what I could manage on my own. My lungs felt like rocks in my chest. I called my husband and he told me to get to the doctor immediately. I had to call back Pastors Patrick and Joy, and was taken to the Military Hospital. Further investigations soon revealed the gravity of the problem.

Clinical examination and X-ray showed that my lungs had collapsed at the right side and there appeared to be pleural effusion (fluid collection at the base of the lungs). This was now an emergency situation, the next 48 hours turned out to be life-threatening. The hospital in Tamale was not equipped to manage the situation and so my office immediately got in contact with the Country Office in Accra for advice. Medical evacuation was clearly needed but the question was; "where would they take me?" We were faced with a dilemma of how best to take me to a hospital that could handle the situation. Air travel was ruled out because the planes available were not pressurized and with low oxygen saturation and no facility for oxygen supplementation, therefore it was not possible for me to travel by air. A shorter road travel of about five hours to Burkina Faso was considered but after discussions with the UNICEF office in Ouagadougou, they felt that the hospital available there may not also be equipped to manage this crisis. The final decision was to evacuate me by road in an ambulance to the Military Hospital in Accra, which had better facilities.

This could not be happening with a major meeting scheduled to take place in a couple of days, I thought as I stared blankly at the faded green coloured wall of the hospital room, this simply could not be happening to me. I soon realized that I had a greater concern to ponder on; knowing the road to Accra as well as I knew the back of my hand, I knew I had trust God to keep me in the hollow of His hands through the journey.

I requested to be allowed to go back home that night, I had no plans of sleeping in that awful room and leaving for Accra without getting back home. The doctor blatantly refused given the gravity of my condition. But, the hospital could not provide humidified oxygen and I had had a bad reaction in the past to dry oxygen supplementation. With the stifling May heat, the hospital room was unbearably hot and stuffy, and the air-conditioner was not functioning. After several consultations and with the consent of my husband, the doctor reluctantly agreed that I would be more comfortable at home in an air-conditioned room and that I needed to have a restful night to face the rigour of the journey ahead the next day. He released me into the care of a nurse from another hospital who by God's divine design had an intensive care qualification.

I was so grateful to God for the opportunity to spend that night at home for a number of reasons. I had to put my house in order and also make arrangements for the care of my young children during my absence. We were not sure how long I would have to be away. I needed to ensure that someone could take care of things in my house should my absence be prolonged, and of course, I had to be sure that the meeting would go on the following morning. My dear family-friends, the Bruce's, were with me for most of the night as I reeled out endless instructions between the coughs and each heavy breath, and handed over all my valuable items. The nurse made me comfortable propped up in bed, but sleep was most difficult, I coughed nonstop throughout the night and all I could do was call on the name of the Lord to keep me. I had no clue what the next few days would be like but I was very sure of one thing, the Lord who brought me thus far and through many of the severe storms in the past, would surely see me through this one. My husband was constantly on the phone, praying with me as we discussed the next course of action.

The Tortuous Road Trip

Prior to my departure on May 6th, 2003, the day my workshop began, I handed my two young sons and their passports to Pastors Patrick and Joy. I asked them to arrange for my children to be brought down to Accra. The white ambulance arrived at my home at 6:00am. I was carefully laid on the propped up couch by the nurse who took care of me through the night and the one accompanying me on the trip. As we drove out of the blue gates, I looked back at my sons, they stood there in front of the house still in their pyjamas — Ose in blue and Ehi in brown—by my pastors and my housekeeper. They looked forlorn, it took them a while to raise their hands and wave at me. "Lord, keep me to see my children again," I prayed with fervency from the depth of my heart. That image stayed with me for a very long time.

> I appreciated the value of family support in the time of illness more than ever before during my stay in this hospital.

The journey to Accra in an Ambulance that had no air-conditioning system and no oxygen was beyond description. Every bump we drove into sent sharp pains deep into my chest. I had insufficient oxygen and was short of air most of the trip. That was the longest trip of my life despite the speed at which the driver was going. I prayed in the spirit throughout the journey. The nurse kept asking me how I was doing. We stopped briefly in Kumasi, about half way through the journey, for the driver and nurse to get something to eat and refuel the vehicle. The two offices (sub office in Tamale and the Country office in Accra) were checking on us as we travelled. We arrived at the Military Hospital ten hours later with the HR officer from the Country Office at hand to receive me. She was stunned when she saw the state I was in. She could not believe the degree of the deterioration in my health since the last week she saw me. I had spent some time with her the previous week.

The hospital staff who received me was shocked that someone in the state I was could have travelled for ten hours without oxygen supplementation. The oxygen saturation was as can be expected, very low. They had been briefed in advance of my arrival, and immediately swung into action as soon as I got there. All I could do was bless the Lord for keeping me with His mighty hands and hiding me inside the hollow of His hands. This was just the beginning of the many wondrous ways God intervened on my behalf during this period.

And She Suffered Many Things of Many Physicians

The next four weeks I spent in the hospital were a testimony of God's mighty deliverance as I suffered many things in the hands of many physicians in the bid to resolve the problem. The enemy assailed me on all sides. Twice the tube had to be inserted into my sides to drain the fluids in my lungs. The pain and discomfort of the intravenous treatment was unbearable. The intravenous line kept failing with the fluid going into the tissue. Both arms were immobilized. I had the blood pressure cuff around one arm, which inflated at regular intervals and the infusion line on the other arm. I was unable to manage food. It was even the more challenging without any immediate family member close by to support me. I was at the mercy of the nurses, until my husband could make it down to Accra. Only the Country Representative and the Chief Operation Officer were allowed to come in once to see me in the High Dependency Unit. I learnt later that several colleagues from the office came but were not permitted in, because visitation was restricted to immediate family only. The loneliness that engulfed me during this period almost drove me to despair. I will expatiate on this later on in this book. Suffice to say, it can be overwhelming to be alone at such a time. I appreciated the value of family support in the time of illness more than ever before during my stay in this hospital.

I did not get on well with the Physician in charge of my care, which was very unusual as I have had very good relationship with my past Physicians. I could not establish a rapport with him. He did not appreciate that I was very knowledgeable about my health situation nor did he like the depth of questions I kept asking. I guess, he was more accustomed to giving instructions to patients who just accepted whatever he had to say. On the one hand, I was very familiar with my medical history. Secondly, I felt he needed to know the details since my case note was not immediately available, especially, when he began to query so many things. I had to request my family back in Nigeria to retrieve my case note from the hospital and send by DHL. I later found that I was screened for HIV without being informed.

There was a brief respite during the period my husband came around. With the stability in the situation, I was moved out of the High Dependency Unit to a private ward. This gave me the opportunity to see my children who had been brought down to Accra a bit more frequently. They were only allowed to see me in the High Dependency ward once and subsequently I saw them through the windows. However, being in a private ward meant that I had to take care of myself most of the time with the nurses only checking in occasionally. Maintenance of hygiene in the room was so poor that I was constantly irritable. In anticipation of an improvement in my health, my husband returned to Geneva to finalise the purchase of our home. We had agreed that I would return to Geneva with the children as soon as I was released to travel. My brother-in-law had to fly in from Nigeria to take care of the boys while they stayed in the hotel, which had become our home away from home during my frequent visits to Accra.

Things took a turn for the worse shortly after my husband departed from Accra, and taking care of myself became more difficult. The doctors discovered that the fluid was re-accumulating in my lungs and I had to undergo another painful procedure to insert the tube into my chest and drain the fluids from my lungs. I was returned to the High Dependency Ward. My husband was unable to come back to Accra at a short notice. The devil assailed my emotions. I was angry and fatigued with everything that was going on. I felt abandoned. It was in this state that my first son's birthday approached. I asked a friend to make a cake for him and then I pleaded with the Matron of the ward to allow the boys and their uncle to visit me. She agreed and I was taken into a small meeting room where I spent some quality time with my son on his birthday.

As a result of the limited improvement in my health, the attending physician proposed a Cardio-thoracic surgery similar to the one I had exactly ten years earlier. He wanted this to be done in another hospital in Accra. I refused to agree to this proposal. I had had enough of the Physician's highhandedness. It was at this time that the UNICEF headquarters approved a medical evacuation to South Africa, which was the country of evacuation for UN Staff based in Africa. However, my husband and I made a special request for this to be changed to Switzerland as this would ensure that I had the much needed family support. The attending Physician opposed the trip. He opined that the surgery could be done in Ghana and he did not think I was strong enough for the travel. I had to exercise my right to a second opinion. I had at this time returned to the private room. I could not have managed by myself there but for the help of a very kind student-nurse who came around occasionally to give me a helping hand; it would have been the last straw on the camel's back for me. The hospital expects family members to be at hand to support the care of the patient. I had none close by. It was so bad that all my underwear were piled up unwashed in a bag in my bedside chest. I kept asking Karen, my Ghanaian friend, each time she visited to bring me new underwear until she asked if I was disposing them. I had to tell her I had no one to wash them for me. I was shocked when she asked me to give the dirty ones to her. She was my gold jeweller who became a very good friend to me. This action on her part took our relationship to another level. She returned the following day with the underwear clean and fresh. She left an indelible mark on my heart.

Against the wishes of the attending Physician, who insisted that a doctor from the hospital must accompany me for the medical evacuation, I opted to be accompanied by a family member. I arranged for my sister to travel from Nigeria to come and accompany me. I needed much help with my personal care and I was not getting that in the hospital. The unhygienic conditions gave me the impetus to request for an early discharge from the hospital two days before I was to be evacuated. The attending Physician and hospital administration refused my request. I was left with no choice but to sign that I was willing to leave against medical advice. I felt I would be better taken care of in the comfort of a clean hotel room by my only biological sister, Mary, who was coming from Nigeria to accompany me on the travel to Geneva. The night I left the hospital, I sat in the bath in the hotel and had a thorough wash. I had never been in such a dire need for a bath in my life. The following day, the doctor and nurse from the UN Clinic came to see me in the hotel. They wanted to ensure that I understood clearly the implications of leaving the hospital against medical advice both for my health and for administrative purposes. They wanted me to be aware that the organisation would be constrained to provide support if I developed any complication as a result of my decision. Secondly, they wanted to ensure that I was stable and in good shape for the travel.

That was when I shared with them the full story of how I had developed bedsores on my buttocks. I told them about my fears that this would get infected because the beddings were not being changed regularly and about the unhygienic state of the toilet. I also felt that I could not report this while I was still in the hospital for the fear of reprisal. I was given emergency numbers to call if I became distressed during the night and the following day before my departure, they promised they would be at hand to attend to me.

Again, it was the mighty hands of God, which held me throughout the flight to Geneva. I was so weak and challenged with breathing that the short walk to the toilet in the plane was an ordeal. I arrived in Geneva with my husband waiting to receive me. He was visibly shaken at my appearance. I had lost over 10kg during my over six weeks stay in the hospital. I was admitted via the emergency room into the Hopital Universitaire de Geneve (HUG) later that day but not before a brief stop at my new home.

#

The Second Surgery On My Lungs

I was first admitted into the general medical ward. They were eight of us in the room with a half drawn screen separating each bed and a large window at the end of the ward. I was farthest from the window and closest to the door. The nurses walked past my bed each time they came into the ward. They soon took note of the incessant coughing, and immediately called the attention of the doctor on duty. Because I was coming from an African country and had an unrelenting productive cough, the first thing the medical team thought of was Tuberculosis. They questioned me about the cough and wanted to know the last time I had the *Mantoux* test—a test to confirm contact with Tuberculosis. Within an hour, I was moved out of the ward and immediately quarantined.

The quarantine room had two wide glass windows. One of them had a speaker I could speak through and answer questions. Nurses and doctors, who came inside were covered in a green overall. They had face-masks on and their hands covered with gloves over the overall. I felt as if I was carrying a plague. Visitors were limited. My family and few friends who were allowed to visit me had to stay on the other side of the glass window. I was like a prisoner in a high security prison talking to my family across the window. No physical contact was allowed. I was kept there until the results of the test for Tuberculosis came back negative.

God in His infinite mercies ensured that the Physician assigned to me spoke English. He was also a very experienced Chest Physician. After reviewing my history and reading through the reports and case notes I brought with me, he called other specialists to join him. This was a complex multi-systemic problem requiring input from multiple experts, he opined. This action proved to be divinely orchestrated in the long run, because it ensured that I was not being passed from one department to the other or with doctors treating a particular disease or system, Prof. PJ was able to coordinate all the other specialists to ensure a holistic approach to my treatment. He will always remain endeared to our hearts for the way he fought for my cause in the coming years.

After several discussions between the team of attending specialists, they concluded that the lungs required immediate surgical intervention. They decided to perform a thoracotomy to remove the fluids that had gathered in my lungs. The pleural lining of the lungs had also become inflamed as a result of all the procedures done during the previous weeks in the hospital in Accra, Ghana.

Exactly ten years after the first surgery on the lungs in 1993, I was back in the theatre again for a second thoracotomy. I woke up from surgery thanking the Lord for bringing me through. However, a few hours later in the recovering room, I was shivering like a leaf tossed by the breeze. The room was dark and cold. I was disoriented. From what appeared to be a long distance, I heard a voice saying there was a drop in my blood pressure. I saw the nurses cover me with a shimmering insulated fabric. I heard the doctors passing instructions to each other as they cut into the blood vessels in my neck. It was as if I was watching them from a distance working on a body. I heard their voices echoing and I could not see clearly. Then, I drifted away into darkness.

When I woke up hours later, my husband was by my side. God kept me through the critical hours and brought me out on the other side. The situation had been stabilized and I was moved to the Intensive Care Unit. I spent a couple of weeks in the hospital recovering from the surgery. After the draining tubes were removed from my sides, the doctors ran a flurry of investigations to help them confirm the diagnosis, before I was finally released to go home.

#

Another New Beginning

Home was the new house my husband and I bought a few months earlier in 2003. I had signed the papers for the house while I was in the High-Dependency Unit in the hospital in Accra, Ghana. I saw the house from the pictures my husband brought along to show me when he visited me in the hospital. The brown coloured outer wall and dark brown wooden front door with our red car parked in front of it was imprinted on my mind throughout my stay in the hospital. I longed to be inside the house. The brilliant white walls, granite spiral stairway and the marble floor in the picture appealed to me. The house fitted my dreams.

When I entered the house for the first time on my way from the airport to the hospital on arrival in Geneva, my mind was too preoccupied and my body too exhausted, to take note of anything but the marble spiral staircase that ran through the four levels of the house.

So it was a great joy to finally step into our home and be introduced to the house properly on that summer day. My sister, Mary, was there taking care of the boys while their daddy shuttled between work and the hospital. Our friends, the Ogundahunsi's were on ground. They stood with us through that season and many more. The entrance level had the guest room, the laundry, a cave and a small lobby leading to the spiral staircase. I knew instantly I was going to have a gilded mirror and a table in that space. The milky marble steps shaped like one-eighth of a circle hung floating from the solid tubular pillar in the middle of the building. Climbing up the spiral steps took us into the sparsely-furnished living room. Sun beams through the sliding glass door flooded the sitting room on the second level making the white walls even more radiant. The glass door was to the right and it opened into the garden bounded by a luscious green hedge on both sides separating us from our neighbours. The outer perimeter was bounded by very tall trees. The garden overlooked a farm across the road. I walked into the garden and looked back into the house and I could see the level above the living room. The house was built to maximize the multi-level topography of the land. Back into the living room, I walked straight into my kitchen at the other end of the living room with the dining room to the right of the kitchen. It had a grey and black marble worktop with butter-yellow cabinets. I never liked small kitchens. I wanted a big kitchen. I had begged my husband to ensure that we have a sizable kitchen, which is a rarity in Swiss houses. I was very pleased with the size of the kitchen. There was enough space to put a freezer and perhaps a small breakfast table.

I made a mental note of what I wanted in each room as we continued the tour of the house. The next level had four bedrooms and a bathroom opening into the hexagonal landing. My bedroom had a bathroom ensuite. They maintained the white walls throughout the house.

"White walls in the boys' bedroom?" I exclaimed. "I will like to see what these walls will look like in a year's time."

"Mummy!!!" The boys protested in exasperation. And we all laughed. It was good to laugh again.

This is home at last. We are all together at home. I postponed the tour of the fourth level to a later date. I was told it has a huge space we can use as a study and also an attic. Very pleased but quite exhausted, I went into my bedroom to rest.

I was totally satisfied with my husband's choice for our home and was ready to begin our new life in Geneva. I was on a paid sick-leave, which we had decided to extend to a Special Leave without Pay on family and health grounds for three months. I needed the time, not only to recuperate from the assault on my health over the past six months and to rest from the stress of my work, but also to support the boys to settle down into their new environment. They started in a new school in September. I knew I would have enough to keep me busy doing up the house.

#

The End of a Chapter In My Life

The three-month Special Leave without Pay came to a rapid end in October 2003. I was much stronger and there had been some respite from the cough. We had an established routine with the boys' school and after-school activities. They needed to have a parent on ground to take them from one activity to the other. The frequency of my husband's work-related travels had become apparent at this time. It became obvious that there was no way I could return to full time work in Ghana while the boys were in school and their father was traveling. We would have to consider either the option of boarding school for the boys, as advised by my professional colleagues, or I would have

> I learnt to depend on God in a new and deeper way when I was stripped of the props and had nothing in the pipeline that could fill the huge vat of needs waiting to be filled at the end of each month.

to stop work and stay back in Geneva—as dictated by my maternal instincts. The boys were already having a lot of challenges settling down in the new school especially my first son, Ose. He was having difficulties making new friends. He had been in four schools in two years and was tired of making and losing friends. Boarding house for them was not an option for consideration. I was at a cross-road and needed to make a choice between my professional career and motherhood.

The lack of salary over the three months was already putting a strain on our finances. We had taken a loan to pay for the twenty percent down payment required for the mortgage of our house from our Credit Union in the US, which we secured with our two jobs and salaries. The loan repayment as well as the mortgage payment had to be accommodated in one salary when I stopped working. In spite of this financial strain, my husband and I agreed that working outside Geneva would not be in the best interest of our family and my still fragile health. We therefore decided that I would extend the Special Leave without Pay for another six months to the end of my contract in Ghana. This was with the hope that I would find another job in Geneva. So I applied and got an approval for this extension of the Special Leave without Pay from the New York Headquarters and I headed back to Ghana in November to close that chapter of my life.

My superiors at work knew the high premium I placed on family. They knew how hard I had argued in the past that women's multiple roles of production and reproduction needs to be recognized by the organization, and women should not have to make a choice between family and career. They were surprised to find me at this cross-road but not surprised to see me choose my family over my career. Some of my colleagues thought it was a rash decision at the brink of my career growth.

"I cannot sacrifice my children's stability for my career," I argued as I tried to convince them. "I need to have my husband and children at my side at the peak of my career development. I don't want to get to the top to find myself alone."

Knowing how much I longed to be a contributing partner in my marriage and also to be financially-independent, my close friends did not think I would last six months without a salary. It was a challenge they were throwing at me and quite honestly, I knew I would need the grace of God to stand up to the challenge.

Upon the completion of the administrative procedures for my extended leave from the organization, and invariably the end of my work in the Ghana Office in Accra, I headed up to Tamale to begin the process of handing over my responsibilities and packing my house. The drive up north was pensive, as difficult and challenging my sojourn in Ghana had been, I had made many great friends and I was going to miss their friendship and the place I had come to know as home in the last two and half years. I spent the entire trip making a list of things to do—both personal and in the office. The list was as long as my arm.

> **I learnt to consciously take a tight rein on my thoughts and command my soul to look only to the Lord and to trust only in God.**

> **The layers of self-reliance, like the dry skin on an onion, were peeled off one after the other until the vulnerable core which would only depend on God was exposed.**

The next few weeks was a flurry of activities; identifying and packing the things I wanted to take back with me to Geneva and giving out the things I no longer needed since my new home came with them. I did not appreciate how much I had grown a family in Ghana until those final weeks. The relationships that I had forged in Ghana tugged my heart as I prepared to leave. There were quite a number of emotional send-off parties organised by my colleagues in the office, the government and non-governmental partners, my church and friends.

Coming to Ghana was God-ordained and for a purpose that I am persuaded will continue to unfold for years to come. The connections I made there will remain dear to my heart. I could not but give praise and thanks to God for the lives He gave me the opportunity to touch for good and for His glory, especially the young couples I mentored. I knew that they will continue to be important parts of my story and my life in the years to come. It was also a preparation ground for fulfilling the call of God on my life. I knew somewhat that the experiences I had during the period were important pieces of the puzzle God is fixing together of my life. He has the picture and each piece is uniquely fitted together. I knew also that I would have to wait with patience for it to unfold in God's good time and in His own perfect way.

> **I knew then that I could not afford to allow my identity to be defined by status, whether professional or financial.**

Perhaps, one day the Lord will give me the grace and opportunity to return back there to share fellowship again with my tribe in Ghana. Until then, I closed the Ghana chapter of my life with praise and thanksgiving to God.

#

Stripped of Props

In earning a handsome salary for over twelve years I had become accustomed to having plenty. I derived pleasure in being able to give generously when asked. My UN job gave me status. Professionally, I was a force to be reckoned with in my field. People listened when I talked and I cannot deny that it felt good. Without any notice, I was stripped of this high profile status that had become an important part of my identity. I spent each day managing our home - cleaning from one level to the other, carting the boys from one activity to another, and overseeing their homework. So many times, I found myself scrubbing surfaces with such intense emotion, pondering what next. Don't get me wrong; I loved being there for my children and

> I learnt through this process that the path to appropriating the fullness of God's blessing is in trustful obedience.

my husband. It gave me joy to be at home when they come back home from school and from work, and to sit on the table with them talking about their day when they chose to talk. But after a while, I began to feel unfulfilled. I missed the spotlight. I missed my incredibly busy agenda. But even above that, I missed the financial independence my job afforded me.

> I learnt to trust and obey God. I learnt to take His Word as is.

Thinking back to when we had major needs in the past years, I could not confidently say I truly trusted God to make provision for that need since I prayed with one eye closed and the other eye gazing on the salary I was expecting at the end of the month. I had one eye lifted to the hills and the other to the props around. I knew no matter how dire the need may be we would be able to work something out at the end of the month.

Prior to my job with UNICEF and in the first few years afterward, my husband and I would make a list of all we needed in the short and long term including capital investments. We prayed regularly over the list and jointly planned the available income while trusting God for His provision. It was always a joy for us to go back and tick off the list as God made a way to get something we trusted Him for. But this began to fall through the crack as we both earned enough to meet most of our needs. And got worse when we had to live in separate locations, therefore managing our accounts separately while still planning major expenditures together and giving each other an account of what we were doing.

I learnt to depend on God in a new and deeper way when I was stripped of the props and had nothing in the pipeline that could fill the huge vat of needs waiting to be filled at the end of each month. It was then, I learnt to rely and lean solely on God as my Provider and my Sufficiency.

It happened slowly. It was subtle, but it was sure, being a contributing partner had become so important to me that I lost sight of trusting God to supply our needs. The financial independence gave me the leverage in decision making and of course, an opportunity for a backup plan. Stripped of a means of contributing, it was hammered home to me that my source of sustenance was not my salary but God who causes us to be supplied and sustained through many channels of which a salary is one. This was when I understood what it really meant that the just shall live by his faith.

We had eight years to pay back the huge loan we took from the credit union in 2003 to secure the mortgage for our home in Geneva, which turned out to be one of the most expensive cities in the world to live in. With our two salaries, we were sure that we would not have any problem paying back the loan as well as paying our mortgage. But we did not anticipate that I would have to come off work three months after signing the contract for the loan and the mortgage because of my health. And when we took the decision for me to leave UNICEF and stay in Geneva with my family, I was very sure that I would find a job in Geneva with one of the UN agencies.

After six months at home with no additional income, my savings became depleted and the monthly repayment of the two loans had to be accommodated within one salary—my husband's. In addition to these loan repayments, we had to accommodate the payment of mortgage, the excess of huge medical bills not covered by the Health Insurance and the children's school fees not covered by the education grant. There were times during that period when my heart raced and my head reeled as the end of the month approached – just thinking about the magnitude of what we needed to pay out.

Every attempt to find a job that would not compromise my health and also give me the much-needed time for my family was abortive. I tried network marketing - Mary Kay Cosmetics, Saladmaster cookware and Herbalife. None of them could give me the kind of additional income we needed but rather was consuming my limited resources to keep up with the demands of network marketing. I did a stint as a volunteer at the

I resolved to confess and speak aloud what I believe.

World Health Organization with the hope that it would give me a foot in the door. But that door never opened to me. And I did not want a travel related job because of my children. At the nick of the time in a desperate situation in 2004, God provided a timely short-term consultancy with an agency. The one-month salary was heaven-sent and then that door closed again.

Several times, my imagination ran riot like a wild horse trying to conjure strategies and map out a way through which God might consider helping us. I thought it would have been great to have a wealthy godfather to turn to, I had none, so I turned to God who is a Father. I wished for a very old and unknown great grand Auntie who would remember us and bequeath a large sum of funds to us, but - it did not happen that way.

Nothing spectacular happened; not for three years. I learnt to consciously take a tight rein on my thoughts and command my soul to look only to the Lord and to trust only in God. It was a period of daily calling upon the name of the Lord and patiently waiting to see how He would come through for us each month. The layers of self-reliance, like the dry skin on an onion, were peeled off one after the other until the vulnerable core which would only depend on God was exposed.

I soon realized how much having a career had defined my identity and I felt somewhat lost without that high profile career. I wonder how many times I asked the Lord why I spent ten years working so hard to get a Doctoral degree only to sit at home or sell beauty products and pots. I had no answer but an assurance that there is a purpose for that season of my life. I knew then that I could not afford to allow my identity to be defined by status, whether professional or financial. Otherwise, I would not see value in my status as a home manager and would devalue the impact my presence at home was making on our family life. It was a struggle indeed. After years of being surrounded by people to give a helping hand with running the house, I had to manage my home singlehandedly for a while.

I must confess and testify that I was overwhelmed by the mysterious ways God worked on our behalf to meet our needs through unexpected and unusual channels. God provided in the most unlikely ways - in His own way, not once in any of the ways I mapped out for Him. He taught me to simply trust in Him and obey His instructions. I had to be quiet to hear Him and I had to be willing to follow His leading.

It reminded me of Naaman; he was introduced as a great man, highly regarded and valiant soldier but he had leprosy. Soon it was obvious that Naaman was also a proud and quick-tempered man, when the man of God did not dignify him with his presence. Only a simple instruction was given; "Go and wash yourself seven times in the Jordan" (2Kings 5:1 – 27). A simple cure was not enough to satisfy him, he wanted a spectacular miracle. Just like him, perhaps I had become proud. Simply living by faith was not enough. I wanted a spectacular miracle for my healing. I wanted a spectacular jaw-dropping miracle of provision.

He was enraged. He felt insulted. His pride was wounded. He resented being asked to wash in an inferior and muddy river like Jordan. I resented not being in control. I resented not being able to spend without counting the cost. I resented not being the high profile 'Mother Christmas' I used to be. Much loved by his servants, they appealed to him as a father to consider obeying the simple instruction. His obedience would require him to be stripped of the strapping of the commander of a great army. He was stripped of the rich and gay clothing covering his leprous body. He was stripped of his pride and prejudice.

His healing would only come if he obeyed the word of the Prophet of God. He humbled himself and obeyed the word of God. As he acted in faith, his body was cleansed. Naaman was healed solely by God's divine grace. I learnt through this process that the path to appropriating the fullness of God's blessing is in trustful obedience. God is often asking for faith and obedience in small matters. Trustful obedience brought abundant water out of a hard rock - a symbol of unyielding hardness.

At that point in my life when I was stripped of affluence, spotlight, and audience, there I learnt to trust and obey God. I learnt to take His Word as is. I learnt to depend on the strength of His promises as if my very next breath depended on it. By the time the spectacular came in 2006, in form of a consultancy provoked by a recommendation from the least expected person, I had learnt to keep my gaze solely on God as my Source and as my Provider. It was a brand new me who packed and headed for another season with UNICEF in Cairo, Egypt. It was a humbled me who had gone to the school of good stewardship that managed the provision from the job which paid off one of the loans. A brand new me whose identity was no longer defined by a high profile job, and affluence but by the God Who called me by my name and had given me influence who took up the new assignment. This experience prepared me for the next phase of my life and the challenges that came with it.

The simplicity of trust and obey in itself magnifies the strength of absolute dependence on God. Now I know what trust means. It is taking God at His word and resting on His promises. It is sweet to trust in Jesus and to take Him at His Word.

**An earlier version of this chapter was published in Effectual Magazine in 2012.*

\#

The Billows Roared

After a period of respite, the billows roared again. It was mid-2005. The events of the previous days demonstrated again that it was the power of God that kept me during the last seven months prior to that day. I came into the hospital for a check-up and found on arrival that I had very low oxygen saturation; I was required to commence oxygen supplementation immediately. After the investigations at the ORL department, the doctors started collecting samples of everything; blood, sputum, urine, faeces etc. The initial results showed that the blood gases were not good. It was agreed that if very good sputum samples could be collected over a period of time, there should be no need for a bronchoscopy and intravenous antibiotics would commence the following day.

> It was only by the grace of God that I regained my confidence while trusting God to bless my intellect with wisdom inspired by the Holy Spirit. I held fast to Him for help at each meeting

The night was bumpy. I got up eventually at 7:00am, prayed a little and had my bath. I became quite breathless after taking the bath with heart racing and pounding in my ears. When the nurses came to check on me about 15 minutes later, they found that the oxygen saturation had dropped again and they put me back on oxygen. I was scheduled to go for a pulmonary function test that morning; it was very difficult and exhausting. While I was having lunch, the ORL Surgeon came to discuss the outcome of the CT Scan and his investigations. He concluded that there was a chronic collection of secretions at the base of my sinuses. He opined that the intravenous antibiotic therapy would not be as effective as it should be if the troublesome bacteria colonizing the sinuses continued to drip backwards into the lungs. He proposed surgical intervention to clean out the sinuses and scheduled the surgery for two days later.

My two attending Chest physicians joined the Surgeon, and confirmed the decision. They both agreed that it was the best way to go. However, they had to discuss with the anaesthesiologist because of the concurrent respiratory problem. The immunologist also came and expressed concerns about how bad things had become over the last seven months. The results so far showed that my respiratory condition had deteriorated over a long time without me paying adequate attention to it. I guessed I just wanted to play down my health issues for a while and not have it as the central focus of our day to day family life. He was amazed how we managed to cope at home without coming into hospital as an emergency. The investigations would have been rushed if it had been an emergency case. He thought it was my resilience and strength but I knew I have been kept by the sheer grace, strength and power of the mighty Hands of God. Watching and listening to the team of doctors discussing the way forward reminded me again of the woman with the issue of blood and how she had suffered many things in the hands of many physicians. Here I was again, surrounded by many physicians just like it was back in 2003.

I recalled how many times things had really been very bad and I slept in the house; how many times the oxygen saturation must have dropped or my heart rate rose to a critical level. I knew like never before that I was kept by the power of God. I meditated on the healing done by Jesus in chapters 4 and 5 of the Book of John in the Bible, when Jesus spoke, things happened and change took place. The child of the prince was restored to life the same hour that Jesus spoke. The rich man believed Jesus and took him at His word. He went home believing and it happened just as Jesus said. The sick man beside the pool at Bethsaida became healed the instant Jesus intervened. Things surely happened when Jesus spoke and it happened immediately. These scriptures assured me that Jesus' word is effective in healing the sick. So I resolved to believe what has been spoken by Jesus in the Bible is effective in my situation as well.

I resolved to confess and speak aloud what I believe;
"I believe in God; I believe He is my Father. I believe Jesus came and died for me. I believe that I am saved. I believe that Jesus is coming back for me. That same faith that effected my salvation is not different from the one I needed to believe that He wants me to be healed and to prosper." And so I began again to lay claim on His Word concerning my life and my healing. God is able to do whatever He wants to do, He does it exceedingly and abundantly above all I could ever dream, desire, ask, imagine and think. He will surely work in His own mysterious ways to perform His wonders in my life.

As I shared the events of the day with my husband later in the evening, it was interesting to note that we came to the hospital when things were getting better or a bit more stable, and not during the critical period we had at home. I saw God's hands in bringing the idea of having the physiotherapy sessions at home to clear the secretions just when the breathing became so difficult at home. That helped to improve the condition of my lungs before we came to the hospital. I understood then how important it was that we came into the hospital without the pressure of the emergency room, which enabled the doctors to coordinate their response properly and yet able to note the severity of the situation. All these made a difference to the plan of action. But more importantly, it encouraged me to keep my focus on God and to continue trusting Him for my healing.

> ———— ✢✢ ————
>
> **I later learnt to turn my times of loneliness to time alone with God.**
>
> ———— ✢✢ ————

A Storm of Gigantic Proportion

The season of storms was not over for the year. I noticed another storm was brewing far in the horizon during the fall of 2005 but I did not anticipate the intensity or impact of the storm until it came ashore. Strong winds of typhoon strength hit me where I was most vulnerable. The gale force winds battered the foundation of everything I held to be true and right. This storm was not like any of the storms we had weathered in the past. This was hitting us at the most unexpected places in our lives. Pain like hot iron seared through the core of my being with each forceful blow of the wind. This terrible storm raged for weeks. But God succoured me in the hollow of His mighty hands and whispered His peace into my hurting heart.

The storm finally subsided. It was in this place of brokenness that healing began. Slowing but surely, we began to rebuild all that was destroyed by the storm. I came out of that storm knowing that the enemy of our soul will stop at nothing to wreck lives in the bid to derail us and ensure that we are not where God wants us to be when He is ready to visit us. I learnt through this storm that unforgiveness is like drinking poison and hoping another will die. I found that God is able to provide the grace to forgive if we are willing to yield our hearts to Him. He can restore what has been broken when we hold fast to His word and wait on Him.

We came out of the storm revived and restored with a resolution to be watchful and on guard against such storms in the future.

#

A Sojourn in Egypt

The sun was blazing in the sky as the plane began its descent into Cairo. I looked down from the window to see the brown sandy landscape. The houses appeared sandy-coloured as we drew close to the International airport. Prior to my arrival, I had read a bit about the city and country. It was my first trip to the Northern region of Africa. The landscape looked somewhat similar to the North-Eastern part of Nigeria. It was October 2006.

I pondered on the trip of Jesus to Egypt as recorded in the Bible and the exodus of Israelites from Egypt via the Red Sea. I hoped I would get to see the Red Sea and play back in my mind how God parted the sea for the Israelites to pass through.

The landing was smooth. Immigration was without any hassle. I collected my huge bags and was met by a driver from the Country Office. I could never have imagined that I would be back with UNICEF again after I separated from the organization in 2004. I was back on a short-term appointment to support the Country's Micronutrient programme. I was excited, but yet filled with trepidation at the thought of re-entering professional life again, this time on my own and with my family back in Geneva. The boys and their daddy would have to take care of themselves for the next six months. Our sons would have to stay with our family friends—the Ogundahunsi's whenever their daddy was away on duty travel. I planned to go back once a month for an extended weekend.

I shifted my focus from my family as we drove through the city. The rickety taxis and the policemen dressed in white uniform caught my attention. I was not quite sure what I was expecting but certainly not the rickety taxis and heavy traffic. The driver was very nice. He gave me a low down about the city and acted like a tour guide pointing out important buildings as we passed them. It was the Ramadan season. Out of the blues, he asked, "Mrs Irene, why do we put on weight during the fast, they told me you are a nutritionist?"

Alright, how do I answer this in a professional manner? I thought.

"Well, you tend to eat more in the night and work less during the day when you are fasting. So you end up not using the calories you consume. You also eat a lot of exotic foods and more fruits, which are not usually a part of your regular diet. Isn't that so?"

He responded in the affirmative and told me how difficult it is for them to work during the day when they are fasting. By this time, we had arrived at my hotel. He deposited me at the Sofitel Hotel in Maadi, which was to be my home until I found an apartment.

It was much more difficult than I anticipated for me to settle down to my position as a Nutrition Expert. I was not feeling at all like an expert. I was no longer sure of myself and as confident as I used to be. I felt I had been a way for too long. I was hesitant to contribute at meetings. I knew I had to quickly commit this feeling to the Lord in prayer. My assignment was challenging enough as it was. I was relating with experts in the field from government and other international agencies and was expected to contribute as an expert. It was only by the grace of God that I regained my confidence while trusting God to bless my intellect with wisdom inspired by the Holy Spirit. I held fast to Him for help at each meeting and He came through for me with the Holy Spirit bringing useful information and facts to my remembrance.

I soon found a thriving Bible-believing church in an Islamic country. Maadi Community Church became my home church. It was amazing that church service was on Friday, the first day of the weekend in Egypt. The service ran with the precision of a Swiss watch. But the content was spiritually uplifting. Before I knew it, I made new friends both at my cell group meetings and in church. I met a Nigerian family in church, and we became bonded together as if we had known each other for ages. Mr K, Tayo and their two sons were strategically located in the place where God wanted me to be connected to them and their friendship proved to be divinely orchestrated and valuable in the course of my stay in Cairo.

Labels of Affliction

It wasn't long before colleagues and partners began to notice the incessant chesty cough and started to make comments about it. "That's a bad cough, are you on antibiotic?" ...and many more comments in the same vein. I was grieved in my heart. The label of affliction had followed me to Cairo as well. The dust and the harsh hot weather were not helpful. Almost all the taxi drivers smoked. The lifts in my apartment building reeked with smoke. Several times I had to tell the drivers taking me on official duties that they could not smoke in the car. This was even more of a concern when I had to go out of town on long distance trips. We would have to stop on the way several times for the driver to smoke. That was quite unnerving for me.

I first heard of the *Haboob* -- sand storm through my colleague and friend in Sudan, who sent me a picture of the one that came over their city. I never thought I would experience it. I was in the office when it was announced that a sand storm was heading towards Cairo. My cleaner sealed every window and door with a masking tape. Notwithstanding all his efforts, I could write a script on the layer of dust on surfaces in the apartment when the storm passed over. I was in a taxi heading to the supermarket late one afternoon when a whirlwind touched down just ahead of us. Soon there was a pillar of dust, dirt and debris making its way towards me as I got down from the taxi. I sprinted into the supermarket and watched the heavy pillar swirl past. I tried to imagine what could have happened if I was caught in the whirlwind knowing the delicate situation of my lungs.

The dust, smoke and heat posed a risk to my delicate respiratory situation. Soon the cough got worse again. I began to have increasing episodes of breathlessness. The cough put more pressure on my bladder and all that went with that. But as if all of these were not bad enough, I started having excruciatingly pain in my abdomen. The severe episodes of bloating made it difficult for me to eat and also limited the space available for my ribs to expand as I breathed.

The more I coughed, the more I got questioned about the cough. I began to confess that the name of Jesus is above every label of affliction the enemy had attributed to me. I confessed the truth of God's word that I have been delivered from every label of identification the Lord did not give me. I declared that all such labels and their influence on my life were broken by the power and authority in the name of Jesus no matter how long they have been associated with me and no matter what purpose they represent.

I was on my way back to Cairo after one of my weekend trips in Geneva in February of 2007, and a hospital check-up as I pondered on these labels. I prayed throughout the trip, proclaiming God's promise over our lives - mine, my husband and my sons. The Lord led me to pray as such as I meditated on Philippians 2 verse 9-11.

In the days following I prayed and trusted in God that every curse that hitherto had held the infirmity in place for that long be broken. I asked God to reveal to me every vulnerable point in my armour through which the arrow of the enemy may penetrate to hurt me. I prayed for an endless flow of strength from God. I knew I had to hold fast to the hope that my healing is assured in Jesus Christ irrespective of the labels of affliction thrown at me.

> I spoke life to myself. I refused to give myself time to feel sorry for me. I chose to focus on the so many things I had to give thanks to God for...

Alone In a Strange Land

My time in Egypt was also marked by times of intense loneliness. It was usually during the weekend. There were times that after coming back home from church on a Friday; I would not get the opportunity for face-to-face adult conversation until Sunday when I returned back to work. I would wait with longing for my husband and our children to call me or be available for my call. There was a weekend that the boys were away on a school trip and my husband was engaged at a conference. I did not get the opportunity to speak to them through Friday and Saturday (weekend in Cairo). I was literally in tears. I was not feeling strong enough to go out of the house. Most of my colleagues had made plans for the weekend and none was available to take my calls. I paced the apartment from bedroom to sitting room. I spent hours by the window watching the sun glowing over the River Nile. I watched the people strolling along Corniche. Soon the sun dropped behind the Sofitel Hotel.

Somehow, I could not shake the feeling of being alone in the whole world that weekend. I wanted to have someone with me in that apartment, someone to talk with face-to-face. That was not possible and I could not even get the opportunity of hearing the voices of family or friends, except for the Arabic filtering through the front door as the children occasionally shouted on the corridor. That was a forerunner of another season ahead of me that I was not yet aware of at that time. I spoke spattering Arabic and could not hold any intelligent conversation with these children even if I had come on the corridor. I begged my husband when I finally got to speak with him, not to let anything get in the way of talking to me during the weekends.

I later learnt to turn my times of loneliness to time alone with God. In His presence, I can never be alone. This lesson proved valuable in the years ahead. But not before I had a rather nasty episode of severe abdominal pain with my tummy so distended that breathing became difficult; even my taking a sip of water, added to the pain. I longed to throw-up the content of my stomach, hoping that it might bring some relief but nothing came out. Yet my tummy was bloated and distended. It was as hard and taut like the top of a conga drum. The pain was beyond description. I lay upside down with half my body on the bed and the other half dangling over a plastic bucket. Still nothing came out. The pain seared through my tummy like a hot iron. I wept like a baby. There was no one around to hear me, comfort me or console me. Fear gripped my heart as I began to ponder on what would happen if I had to call for help. There would be no way for anyone to gain access into the apartment to help me except if they broke down the wall. I did not even know who would be the appropriate person to call in case of an emergency

I made it a point of duty to ask as soon as I got to work the following day. Yes, the pain did pass. The distension went down a bit and I got some relief before the night was over.

In A Vicious Cycle

The cough became vicious again in late July 2007 as it became more frequent and intense again. This was probably the third or fourth episode of chest infection at that scale that year. I got very concerned when I saw the colour of the secretion, it was becoming dirty again. A cry welled up in my heart, "I am not going through this vicious cycle again." Has God not promised me that affliction will not come upon me a second time? Why then does this affliction keep rearing its ugly head? The life-giving breath of God and disease causing agents cannot cohabit in my lungs, when light comes in darkness must recede. When life flows in, sickness and death must recede. I began to pray that the fire of the Holy Spirit will consume once and for all every strain of pseudomonas in my lungs, in my sinuses and in my body. I declared that every pathogen and disease causing agents that had taken residence in any cell of my body be destroyed in the power and authority that is in the Jesus name.

I was honestly tired of the several courses of antibiotic therapy I have had. And the resultant effect on my tummy. I would have to go back to Geneva for the intravenous antibiotic treatment, which would usually last for twenty-one days. That was a time I could not afford to spare. I could not accumulate leave days since my monthly trip to Geneva required that I take two leave days every month for the extended weekend.

The weather had become hot, severe and harsh at this time and it was the same story with the project I was working on in the office.

A Tornado Touched Down

For a project that took off remarkably well and maintained its course with no major bump, we were unprepared for the crisis that developed in the last phase of the work. The unexpected came roaring and twisting like a tornado and touched down on the project and in the lives of everyone closely associated with it. In what appeared to be a twinkling of an eye, the project spiralled off its axis. The sudden swift twist left me giddy. The ensuing crisis strained my skills in advocacy and diplomacy beyond its limits. This project was the centre-piece of my work in Cairo. It was a national project. I had worked in very close collaboration with government partners who had come to respect me over my almost a year sojourn in the country. I had developed a very close relationship with a few of them while implementing the project. Whatever else that I did well in the country would pale in significance if I was unable to stir the project to its logical conclusion.

The interim report produced by the external facilitator—an esteemed senior colleague was rejected outright by all the government partners. From this point on, everything that could go wrong went wrong. Every day presented with new set of problems and more difficulties to the extent that some people opined the project was jinxed as those immediately associated with it suffered one personal calamity after the other, which further hindered them from fulfilling their assigned roles. My respiratory problem had grown worse in the heat and humidity of the summer month.

Frustrated, desperate and feeling like my back was against the wall, I went to church. One of the worship songs was Graham Kendrick's "To You O Lord." The few lines I could remember resounded in my heart all the way back home—as if that was all I heard in church that day. It tugged at my heart and I knew I had to find the full lyrics. I searched the Internet, found it and the scripture it was based on - Psalm 25. I meditated on the entire passage and the song. The first three stanzas became the rock upon which I anchored my prayers as I entreated God concerning the project.

"O Lord, in You do I put my hope, let me not be put to shame. My eyes are on You."

Those who put their trust in God will never be put to shame so I set up my computer at work to play the song continuously to remind me throughout the day to persist in prayers and to trust that it is only God Who could make a way for me through the wilderness. I remembered again that I was in Egypt. God made a way through the Red Sea for

I must keep reminding myself that this must be to the glory of God. Not because I wanted it to be me doing it but God's purpose being fulfilled in people's lives through the things He allows me to be a part.

the Israelites to be delivered from the hands of their oppressors. I knew He would deliver me by His mighty and outstretched hands just as He did in the times of old.

There were moments when I panicked and allowed myself to picture what it might look like if we could not complete the project. The picture frightened me. I knew we could not afford to fail - it was not an option, and I could not afford to give up on the hope of finding a solution to the problems.

"Oh Lord I need You. Remember me according to Your mercy and love."

I needed divinely inspired wisdom and insight to get the lead team to work together, to have the entire report rewritten and ensure ownership by the primary stakeholders without compromising the already fragile and tense relationship with the external team. It was at this time that I went back to Geneva for my regular check-up. The past weeks had been extremely challenging at work. The weather was most unfavourable and my health was deteriorating. I needed to see my doctor.

Needless to say, it was a double tornado that had touched down. I was standing precariously at the edge of the cliff with my health. My blood gases were deranged and oxygen saturation had become too low to the extent that the poor respiratory condition was putting a strain on my heart. It was overworking. My doctors told me the only solution was for me to be on a continuous oxygen supplementation. My heart fell like a rock within me. How was I going to continue working in Cairo on oxygen supplementation? This was the question plaguing my mind. I was told that the only condition under which my doctors were willing to consider allowing me to return to Cairo was if I could confirm that supplemental oxygen will be available for my use both at home and in the office when I returned to Cairo.

I cried to the Lord for help and in His mercy, He hearkened to my cry.

God sent help. The family, God had raised up for me as friends in Cairo, agreed to help me look for an oxygen concentrator for the house and a cylinder for the office. With the support and help of my Chief of Section, the Country Representative and Chief Operation Officer agreed for me to have the oxygen cylinder in the office. It was with this assurance that my doctor gave me the medical certificate that allowed me to travel back to Cairo. I had an unfinished assignment to complete in less than three months. It would take God's direct intervention to make that happen.

My friends, the Kupoluyis, had their driver waiting for me on my arrival back to take me to their house, after I had completed the 21-day course of intravenous antibiotic treatment in Geneva. Not only did they provide all I needed but they refused to allow me to go and stay in an apartment alone. I stayed in their home for the rest of my sojourn in Cairo with my girl-friend watching over me with eagle eyes.

Against the odds, we constituted a smaller team to finalise the project. The three of us had stories to tell of the calamities that befell us during the last six months leading to that time. We worked with a renewed resolution that we would not be defeated. We worked tirelessly day and night to rewrite the entire report until it was acceptable both to the Government partners and the international community. Many times during the meetings, I would rush down to my office to spend some precious time refilling my lungs with oxygen while praying and asking God for direction.

At the presentation of the results to the scientific community, my co-presenter and one of the lead facilitators of the project openly declared that the project came to a successful conclusion simply because of perseverance and patience. To these I added - persistent prayer anchored on hope that does not disappoint.

Faced with the possibility of failure, I needed a relentless determination not to give up on the hope in the miraculous ability of God to bring deliverance in Egypt and in the wilderness of life. God turned what was seemly a hopeless situation around in a way that even the heathen affirmed that it was the hand of God working on my behalf. There was no other way to explain the grace He caused to abound to me to sustain me despite my failing health through that storm or the remarkable support and help He raised for me through people I never knew before I came to Egypt.

My contract came to an end at the end of December with my assignment successfully completed. My husband and sons joined me for Christmas. Together, we wrapped up my sojourn in Egypt. For the second time, I exited UNICEF on health grounds at the brink of a promising career. I had no regret. I went to Egypt for a purpose. That purpose had been accomplished and included was the bonus of paying off a significant proportion of our debts.

I returned to Geneva on January 8th, 2008 to give focused attention to my health. Another chapter of my life ended when I boarded that last flight out of Cairo. I left behind great friends and left with great memories.

\#

Riding the Waves

It was not the big waves that moved me, it was the small waves. I sat calmly as the doctor told me of the possibility for me to have to consider a lung transplant. You would have thought they told me about getting an X-ray done. I was unmoved and unshaken. I had peace in my heart. I needed a new pair of lungs and I know God has it in store for me. But when my oxygen cable got stuck under the doorway on the way to the bathroom, I got really angry and frustrated with having to live with this cable. The cable always seemed to get stuck under the bathroom's door way, such that as I got to the toilet and I wanted to sit, it stopped short and jerked me back. It was very annoying especially when I was rushing to the bathroom with a full bladder. I found it very frustrating not being able to do all the things I had on my list to do. Sometimes, it was just so difficult to get small things done. It took so much effort, I was breathing like someone who is running a marathon just to have a bath, or arrange things, or go shopping. And I love to shop. Imagine not being able to go to the shops, which is my stress management exercise, simply because I could not handle it or not being able to cook up something in the kitchen because I just did not have the strength to do so.

> My words echoed in my ears and I knew in that instant that I had spoken the wrong words into existence. So I cried out to God to forgive me.

So how could I, who seemed to calmly ride the big waves, find it so difficult to deal with the small waves. Sometimes I looked at myself in the mirror and I saw the strained look on my face from the effort it took to breathe or trying to catch my breath, it is so difficult not to feel sorry for yourself, but I have learnt to talk to my image in the mirror and speak life to it.

"God is the giver of life and breath, He is the sustainer of life and breath. He is the sustainer and maintainer of my life. I have life and I have it more abundantly". I spoke life to myself. I refused to give myself time to feel sorry for me. I chose to focus on the so many things I had to give thanks to God for, especially the grace He gave me not to dwell in self-pity. I thank God for that grace. One thing I knew was that every bit of this process of healing would be used of God for His own purpose and for His own glory.

I have found that music does a lot to help me deal with the situation and stay focused on God. There were so many songs that God used to minister to me and to lift my spirit up. Some of the lyrics are so rich that they were imprinted on my heart. God used diverse ways to provide stability for our soul when we are faced with challenges and very difficult situations. He stills the agitations these events tend to bring. He carries us above the waves. We can ride above the big huge waves and the small waves in Him.

#

Taking Notes: He Would Not Ignore Me

It was in May of 2008 that I started writing again to chronicle my experiences, the events of my life and all the things I believed the Lord was laying on my heart that had been an encouragement to me. I had much flowing through my heart that I wanted to write down. I was not sure I would be able to get all of them on paper, but I decided to keep trying. Procrastinating meant that I would not remember them again and would have lost a valuable opportunity of putting down things that were helping me to deal with the situation, which could also help others.

One morning I remembered an old song. I thought it must be in the Methodist Hymn book. I could only remember the last line in Yoruba - "*Baba kio fi omo re si le ko sokun lai nidi.*" Literally translating that, it means, A father will never watch His child cry for no reason or He will never leave His child alone to cry for no reason. That ministered to me in many more ways than I could describe. If my earthly father will not stand aside and watch his child suffer for no reason, then I was persuaded that God will not just stand aside and watch me suffer for no reason. There is a purpose and reason for what I was going through at that time. There is something God was building in me; there is something I was being shaped for. And in the fullness of time, God will make it manifest... I told myself.

One of our senior friends from UCH, Ibadan, Prof W. came to Geneva for a conference and he stayed with us. During his stay, he shared something with me that connected some dots for me. He used the same verses God ministered to me earlier that week as he prayed with us. He asked me if it was recorded in the Bible that there was anyone Jesus could not or did not heal. I had not read anywhere in the Bible where Jesus did not heal those who came to Him. I knew very well also that God wants me to be healed, He desires for me to be healed. Healing is my portion in Christ Jesus. He has blessed me with every spiritual blessing in heavenly places in Christ. He has given to me all that pertains to life and godliness. He promised me that He will not put upon me any of the disease He put on the Egyptians. How He does it or when He would do it are questions that I could not begin to labour on. One thing that I knew for sure was that if God says He has healed me then I am healed. He is the Lord that heals me. It does not matter whether what I am seeing or feeling is contrary to that promise. That promise holds true irrespective of all that was. I had to know in all my knowing that God was working out something in me through this illness that will be used to His own glory.

I chose to keep praying. I chose to stay with the word and hold fast to it.

I knew I have a story to tell. I believed that God is preparing me to tell my story. But when that story is to be told and to whom the story is to be told, I really did not know. Only God knows that. There is a way you feel as if you are going to bust if you do not tell the story. But I did not want to do my own thing. I had to wait and go through the preparation. The story needed to be processed in the way God wanted to use it. It is also God who is preparing those who need to hear the story. At His appointed time and place, He will bring those who need to hear in contact with the story, so that His will can be fulfilled and He will get all the glory. In the interim, I must patiently go through the processing so that I will truly be used of God to do what He wants me to do. I was certain that the story will unfold in due course when the time is right.

The Bible says that the vision is for an appointed time. We are to write it down and make it plain, so that they that read it can run with it. I decided I was going to keep writing the story down as it unfolded.

With the renewed desire to write, I was determined to get out of bed earlier than my usual time and start my routines early. I wanted to spend quality time writing my entries. There was so much to catch up on and I did not want to miss out on the new things that the Lord was ministering to me. I spent a bit of time ruminating on my heart desires, my dreams and the vision I carried in my head for my life. I will share some of them below:

> And He heard my cry and came through for me. The storm subsided, and the tranquillity was music in my ears as I finally slept off.

- I desire to be God's finger tips touching lives
- To add value and make a difference to the lives of everyone I come in contact with
- To be the bearer of God's answer/ miracle to someone's prayer
- To be a conduit of God's blessing
- To be God's handmaiden
- A woman who honours the Lord
- To be able to enrich peoples' lives in so many different and unique ways
- I desire that God will make me a Masterpiece, an instrument, a song of praise and for Him to put me on display.

I dreamt of the many ways I could fulfil these goals and desires. I often allowed my imagination to run "riot" just thinking up things I could do in the service of the Lord. I love to inspire people; I love to give people a reason to be hopeful. I just love to impact people's life positively. But I must keep reminding myself that this must be to the glory of God. Not because I wanted it to be me doing it but God's purpose being fulfilled in people's lives through the things He allows me to be a part. I acknowledged and kept upfront in my heart and head that whatever I desire to do must be in partnership with God and for His glory only. I knew I must never share God's glory. NEVER!

So I laid in bed for a while, thinking about all of these. I wondered how it would come to pass. I was assured by God that the vision was for an appointed time, it would surely come to pass but for now I must patiently endure the process that prepares me to be used of God to fulfil His purpose for my life and His purpose in the lives of others. There was a lot going on in my head that morning about keeping hope alive, not giving up, and staying with the vision. There was also a lot about not running ahead of God but waiting for God's appointed time. After spending sometime praying, I wanted to study something that could help me build up my faith and to keep hope alive. I opened my Bible to Hebrew 11 and I was really blessed.

My desire is to fulfil God's purpose and plans for my life, to enter into the fullness of His promises for me. The foundation of my hope and desire must be fixed on God. The plans for my life are His. The purposes for my life are His. The appointed vision, goal, accomplishments are His. He is the architect of my life and He only can build me up to fulfil and fit into His plans and purposes for me.

My hopes and desires must be in Him. I cannot find fulfilment outside His eternal and divine purpose for my life. Whatever I desire to do and to be must be fitted within His divine purpose for me to have true fulfilment.

Knowing that also gave me hope and another level of understanding because all I was passing through right then were not purposeless, they were being used by God to shape me, prepare me and make me ready to be what and who He wants me to be.

He knows the thought He thinks towards me, thoughts for my good, to give me a hope and a future, and to bring me to a perfect and expected end. His thoughts for me are thoughts that bring me good, they are good thoughts. He desires to give me hope, something to hope for, something to hold unto, something to wait expectantly and with confidence for. He had seen ahead. He knew I needed such an anchor to hold me steadfast. He has a future for me, an assured future. He has a perfect and expected end for me, a perfect end for me when I would hear Him call me; "Thou faithful servant."

I do have a life worth living and a hope worth keeping alive. Jesus died to give me a life worth living. So I purposed in my heart to hold on. I purposed in my heart not to give up. I gave my desires and dreams wings of hope. Faith cannot act in a void. Faith is based on hope. There is something to hope for out of my current situation. I have a hope. My faith is the assurance, the conviction, the reality of the things that I hope for which I have not yet seen.

#

Almost Gave Up

If there was one time that I almost gave up on the struggle, it was in November 2008. But God kept me. He held fast to me. I felt I could not take one more day of the pain. I felt I could not take one more bout of that horrible cough. I got tired of struggling for breath. I was fed up with not being able to lift my head without feeling fatigued and exhausted. I got tired of life the way it was, and I voiced it.

Things were really bad at this time. I felt it was simply too much for me. I began to wonder if the time to go home to be with the Lord was drawing nigh. I began to search my heart to see if there were persons I was holding bound there. Those who offended me and I had yet to release from my heart. I asked God to forgive me for not forgiving and letting them go from the prison of my mind. I made efforts to settle with those I thought I might I have hurt. I was not ready to miss heaven because I was harbouring offenses, bitterness and unforgiveness in my heart.

I made a list of all I own, my jewellery, head-ties and stuff that I thought I would like to bequeath to my family and friends. I made a mental note of who I wanted to have what. During the conference, I was having with the 'board members' in my mind—those voices that bring all manner of suggestions. I wrote my will. I even decided what I wanted to be given to my daughters-in-law when they come as my gift to them. I knew I had to be able to place the fat yellow notebook where the instructions and list were made where my husband will eventually see it. The 'board members' made quite some appealing suggestions. That is their major pre-occupation—to make suggestions, and often not by the Spirit of God.

I was still in consultations with the 'board members' when I had to go into the hospital to see my doctors. It was becoming increasingly difficult to hold air in my lungs. My body was demanding more oxygen. I was admitted to the short-stay ward. That night, I voiced the suggestions of the 'board members'. I actually put into words and told a dear and respected sister who called me from Nigeria to check on me; "I am tired." It was technically true. But this phrase went forth with power to call forth a thunderstorm. I knew as soon as the words left my mouth that something shifted. I felt it in my spirit but I did not pay attention to the urgent stirring. I did not retract my words. They almost proved fatal!

By the following morning, the oxygen saturation dropped to such a low level that the short walk from the bed to the bathroom caused my head to reel and darkness enveloped me. I could not leave the bathroom. I called for the nurses. From there on, I went downhill. Because of this rapid deterioration in my respiratory functions, the doctors moved me to the high dependency ward. I had the electrodes stuck on me and was being monitored closely. My husband came to see me there that morning. After he left, my condition deteriorated further. Before he had the chance to get back to the office, my doctors took the decision to move me to the Intensive Care Unit. Prof. PJ had to call him back to the hospital.

The strong forceful winds of the storm swirled me around violently. I stared down a deep dark vortex as if I would drop or be sucked into it. Then I saw what I knew to be the finger of God looking like a hook holding the back of my neck over the deep pit - close your eyes and imagine your shirt hanging on a hook behind a door. That was how I felt hanging over that pit with

God's finger holding me from falling headlong into it. God kept me. He didn't let go of me.

My words echoed in my ears and I knew in that instant that I had spoken the wrong words into existence. So I cried out to God to forgive me. He did and He was already holding me back from being sucked into the abyss.

Physically, the event unfolding was intense. My doctors determined that my lungs were becoming too weak. I needed non-invasive ventilation, but every equipment tried did not work. I could not manage the pressure of the ventilators. I felt like someone drowning in the deep sea with each one we tried until they brought the one that looked like the helmet of astronauts on the way to outer-space. The technician placed it over my head and they began to regulate the pressure until breathing felt right again.

I decided that I would take His Word like my medicine. His Word is life to me, healing and medicine to my flesh.

I saw the image of myself reflecting from the window to the Nurses' bay across my bed. My head was encased in the round transparent helmet with an airtight collar around my neck. There was a small window on the helmet through which I was given drinks via a straw and my drugs were administered. The image was unnerving.

I knew I must fight for life. I must determine to see the goodness of God in the life of the living. There were several reasons for the fight for life. Top on the list was the desire to be here for my husband and to see my sons become the fine God-fearing men I know God has created them to be. I wanted to be here to see the goodness of God manifesting in their lives. I could not afford to give up on life.

#

The Valley of Affliction and Pain

The special song the choir sang in church on Sunday April 27th, 2009 resonated with my spirit. It was "We Will Remember" by Tommy Walker. The third stanza anchored itself deep within my heart that day and remained my companion for many years later.

"When we walk through life's darkest valleys
We will look back at all You have done
And we will shout our God is good
And He is the faithful one

Chorus:
We will remember we will remember
We will remember the works of Your hands
We will stop and give You praise
For great is Thy faithfulness

I was careful not be angry or become resentful. I realised that I would have to release this case into God's hands and let it go.

I sang the chorus repeatedly, and ruminated on the lyrics. By the evening of the same day, the enemy began an onslaught of attacks. I had a nasty episode of allergic reaction that resulted in severe bronchospasms over the next few days. I lost count of the number of times during that day I cried out, "Please help me, I can't breathe."

From that time on, it was one attack on my health after the other to the extent that I could not go to church for the next three Sundays. The enemy of my soul assailed me on all fronts. I had a rather painful sprain on my hand on top of all that was going on making it difficult to hold things. The last straw was on the Wednesday of the third week of the onslaught of attacks when I started having a horribly excruciating pain in my stomach. It was so bad the following day that I could not sleep throughout that night.

I quoted and confessed all the healing verses I knew. I wept. I wailed. I cried. I shouted to the Lord out of my distress. It felt like the intensity of the pain of a woman in Pitocin-induced labour with no rest or respite between the contractions. I know how that feels I had been there before. This pain brought back the memories of that fateful day in January 1993, when I cried out in agony not only from the pain of the Pitocin-induced labour but out of the sorrow searing deep into my heart. I was delirious with pain by Friday morning. The worst part of it was that I could not scream. I had guests in house. I had children in the house. It reminded me so much of Hausa ladies I met in the labour ward while conducting the research for my Masters' degree. While all the other ladies were screaming at the top of their voices, these ladies simply held fast to the bed post, gritting their teeth and breathing hard. You would hear them moan softly during the final stages of the labour but never a scream. I had to do the same thing each time the waves of pain engulfed me and if felt as if a hot knife was piercing through my tummy. I too held fast to my bed pane and breathed hard. When it passed, I began to speak the word of God to my body. By noon of that Friday, all I could say was, "Lord, please take this cup away from me. Please make it go away."

Gosh! There is just some kind of pain that is beyond words. I had been through some of this kind of intense pain in the past. I recalled a time when I had the same kind of pain in my tummy. I had just completed a 21-day course of intravenous antibiotic treatment, which somehow messed up my tummy. I became bloated. It was so bad that I had difficulties breathing. The home-nurse called in an emergency doctor who insisted that we must call in an ambulance. I could not imagine having the noise of the siren in my quiet neighbourhood and the ambulance in front of my house. I felt it would announce to all my neighbours that something was wrong. I told the doctor that I would prefer my husband drove me to the hospital. He eventually agreed and my husband took me to the hospital. We got to the emergency room and it took over six hours for the nurse to put me on a couch. It was when I fell on the floor writhing in pain after almost six hours of sitting and waiting that the nurse eventually put me on a couch to await the attending doctor. Priority attention was only given to patients brought in by the ambulance. That was when I understood why the doctor had insisted on calling the ambulance. My husband was very upset at the ordeal I had to go through because we went in by ourselves. I swore I would never go the Emergency room by myself again.

I had a similar experience with this kind of pain while I was in Cairo. It was all through the night. At a stage, I got very worried because I lived there alone. I wondered how anyone would get to me in my room even if I called out for help. The door had a security barricade behind it. I knew that it was only God who could help me at such times. This was one of those times. Little did I know then that these would all pale in significance to what was coming in the years ahead.

Then as if the devil got angry, the pain got worse on this Friday afternoon. Finally, I decided that I would have to call my doctor if the pain did not stop by 3:00 pm. Perhaps, he would be able to do something to stop the pain but I knew he would definitely ask me to call the ambulance. The pain had gone on for three days. I had come a long way with it. I did not want to go to the hospital. The International Day in my sons' school was scheduled for the following day. I had promised them that if I could not go with them, I would at least cook some Nigerian dishes for them to take to school. I had missed so many of their school activities. I did not want to disappoint them again on this one. My husband was also scheduled to travel on Sunday. Going to the hospital on Friday was not an option. It was bound to disrupt all the family plans for the weekend. My husband would not be able to travel with peace of mind if he had to leave me in the hospital.

I shared all my concerns with God and pleaded my case. I asked Him to stretch His mighty hands and pluck me out of the deep valley of affliction. I asked Him to speak peace to the turbulent storm of pain. I held fast to the word and continued to confess what the Word of God said about my healing. I latched relentlessly to hope. I clung to God's unfailing promises. And He heard my cry and came through for me. The storm subsided, and the tranquillity was music in my ears as I finally slept off.

By 7:00pm, I was able to come out of my room and down to the living room. And by 8:30pm, I was in the kitchen cooking. By the time the boys and their dad left for the International day at noon on Saturday, I had finished cooking three different dishes, which they took with them for the show. After they all left, I dropped on the sofa tired but feeling victorious. Who would have thought that barely 24 hours ago I could not get out of bed let alone talk of making three dishes? Who would have imagined 24 hours ago that I would not be on the hospital bed at that time?

Truly the enemy came against me from all fronts yet the Lord gave me the grace to fight back. The enemy assailed me like the way my son described the way girls fight — they use everything they've got. They kick. They bite. They scratch. The picture is even more vivid when they are fighting an older, bigger and taller brother. But it is only a matter of time before the stronger brother subdues the clawing and kicking little sister. That picture imprinted on my heart what my Father, the Mighty Man of war together with hosts of heaven did on my behalf. Though the enemy kicked, clawed and swung his fist at me, when the Lord God rose up on my behalf, he was speedily subdued. As I pondered on the events of the past three weeks, I remembered again the song we sang that Sunday in church three week earlier. I started singing that song, and this one was written by Reuben Morgan (Integrity Hosanna Music). I sang these songs with the joy of one who had come out on the other side of the valley victorious;

> "I'll walk closer now on the higher way
> Through the darkest night will You hold my hand?
> Jesus, guide my way
> Oh, You mourn with me and You dance with me
> For my heart of hearts is bound to You
> Though I walk through valleys low
> I'll fear no evil
> By the waters still my soul
> My heart will trust in You
> Though I walk through valleys low
> I'll fear no evil
> By the waters still my soul
> My heart will trust in You
> My heart will trust in You

Oh, You counsel me and You comfort me
When I cannot see, You light my way

Though I walk through valleys low
I'll fear no evil
By the waters still my soul
My heart will trust in You"
(Hillsong – My Heart Will Trust)

My husband and I looked back that night to the three weeks that had passed, and we saw what God had done; the deliverance He had again wrought for us. All we could do was shout that our God is good and He is the faithful one. My husband left on duty travel the following morning with peace in his heart, being fully persuaded that the Lord was able to keep me. It was amazing and we could testify of all that the Lord revealed to us in that deep valley of affliction. He reminded us of many unfinished businesses that we needed to deal with — stuff we were holding on to in our hearts that we had to let go of. He confirmed some of the things He had spoken to us in the past. He brought us in contact with messages that ministered to us just where we needed it. And He put the icing on the cake and brought us specific friends who committed themselves to stand in the gap interceding for us in prayers.

We will still have more reasons to remember the works of God's mighty hands in our hands. After each valley of affliction experience, we always can look back and praise God who sustained us and brought us through it victoriously.

#

Life in the Word and in a Name

It was the 23rd day of October, 2009, I considered what God had done throughout that year and I knew truly that *Oluwadamilola* - God looked upon me to favour me. I was back in the hospital. Coming out of the toilet into the room I was given and noting the number of times I had to go to the toilet because of the pressure the heavy cough put on my bladder, I felt so overwhelmed at the awesome love and kindness of God in blessing me with the room.

Though the stay in the Rolle Hospital at this time was pre-planned for a time when the doctors felt I would be physically strong enough to benefit maximally from the rehabilitation, I started feeling quite poorly the week before my admission. I was coughing a lot again, secretions increased with the worrisome colour, and I felt very tired and more breathless. It happened so rapidly, that by the weekend I had had a couple of days of chills and fever. I was upset that all these were happening again barely one month after the last intravenous antibiotic treatment.

I told my husband that the effects of the last treatment seemed to have lasted for only one month, and he quietly told me that his trust was not in the treatment but in the Lord. Truly our trust is in the Lord, and those who put their hope and trust in the Lord shall not be moved but like mount Zion shall abide forever. I have a hope that makes not ashamed, a hope that does not disappoint. I am persuaded that we have seen the end of this thing. Though many are the afflictions of the righteous man but surely the Lord delivers me from ALL of them, He healed me from every one of the diseases that hitherto afflicted me.

The hospital had called me on Tuesday morning to alert that they did not have a private room for me. The available shared room also had no shower or toilet, which meant that I would have to go down the corridor each time I needed the bathroom. Mindful that we were pressured for time with my husband's forthcoming duty travels I accepted what they had to offer.

When Dr. J-PC came on a home-visit later that day, he was not happy at my state of health especially at the rapidity of the deterioration. He did not feel it was a good time to go to Rolle and he confirmed that I needed again the intravenous antibiotic therapy. He wanted a consultation with the specialist and proposed that Rolle be rescheduled until following week while I commenced treatment at home. He was also concerned about the risk that I might be exposed to if I have to share a room with someone with an infection, and I may also pose a risk to others.

The following Wednesday I got a call from the doctors to go to Rolle as planned on Thursday, and that all that was needful would be done there. On arrival in Rolle, not only did they have a private room for me, it also had its own toilet and shower. The enormity of God's favour in giving me this facility became obvious as I frequently needed to use the bathroom and this would have posed a challenge as I would have had to change from the main Oxygen supply to the portable Oxygen each time I had to go outside the room to use the bathroom. It was convenient being able to get up from the bed and to walk straight into the toilet, being so

> **As I recalled the deeds of the Lord and called to remembrance His wonderful miracles of old, His peace flooded my heart.**

fatigued already I could do without the added stress. I would have been unable to handle rushing to the bathroom when under pressure.

Having Peter and the boys with me at this time was important to me. It would have been difficult for them to stay a long time and for us to spend time together as a family if I had to share a room with someone else. It is this family time that helped me get through the ordeal of long hospital stays. I looked forward to their visits and the boys goofing around me. With my usual stream of visitors especially from the church, being alone in the room gave us the opportunity to pray together without disturbing anyone.

In summary I saw the hands of God working on my behalf, such that if I must be at the hospital it was made comfortable and bearable for me. God is truly worthy of our praise: *Oluwatosin* - my middle name.

The rapid re-occurrence of the infection was of grave concern to the doctors too, who felt that there might be loss of sensitivity to the drug being used and with the reducing period between each treatment, they needed to reconsider using the same drug again for the fourth time that year. The bug colonising my lungs was becoming resistant to the drug of choice.

I decided that I would take His Word like my medicine. His Word is life to me, healing and medicine to my flesh. And it can never lose its sensitivity nor can the affliction become resistant to it. A Word from Jesus and the sick were restored to health. He sent His Word and it healed me. Surely, His Word will not return to

Him void but it shall fulfil the purpose for which it has been sent in me. So I determined to pay attention to confessing the word of God and His promises concerning me over the situation. I began to feel full of life in my being as I received the life-giving power in God's word. There is life in the word of God that is poured into my body as I speak and confess the Word over my life.

It was while meditating on using the Word of God as my medicine that the following questions began to filter into my spirit. "How can a man die being so full of life?" and "How can I die so full of life?" As a child of God, I am supposed to be full of the life of God. I knew from the Word of God that I have the life of God in me. So I began to confess that "I am full of life, vitality and energy. I have the fullness of life in me. The Word of God dwells in me in all its fullness.'

My husband told me repeatedly that we don't have to be religious with God. We can tell Him how we feel and He will respond to us in the way that will best minister to us.

I bless the Lord who gives me life to the full and running over. Despite going to sleep late, even in the hospital, and having intravenous treatments at 12:00 midnight and 6:00am, I still slept with an indescribable feeling of peace and calmness. It almost felt unusual. The usual distress and feeling of harassment that I experienced whenever I went on the ventilator was not there at all. I woke up one morning with such a feeling of fullness of life that I had to note it down. The oxygen saturation was 91 at 3L that morning, the best record since I got there. God is worthy of our praise - *Oluwatomisin*.

#

It Is Payback Time

Earlier that year in June 2009, I spent several days listening to some teaching by Joyce Meyer, and I read a number of scriptures from the Bible and a book that gave me reasons to consider adding another dimension to my praying. There were a couple of people who owed me for things they purchased from me a few years back. One of them had blatantly refused to respond to all the overtures I made during the year to get her to pay up. So many times I had asked the Lord what to do. As I listened to Joyce Meyers, she spoke about trying to collect from someone who cannot pay you back. Well, I thought that is not applicable to this particular case, because there was a time this individual could not pay me back and during that period I did not ask her about the funds. But now it does certainly appear that she was in a better situation to consider paying me what she owed but she avoided my calls and did not respond positively. I was careful not be angry or become resentful. So when I picked up the book by Joel Osteen and there again it was written, to let the Lord right the wrong that had been done me and not to try to collect from someone who does not want to pay me back. I realised that I would have to release this case into God's hands and let it go. I must trust God will pay me back abundantly.

I recalled the many times things were stolen from me. I was in the hospital with no immediate family around to hand my valuables over to, so I kept them with me. Only to discover one day, despite keeping them where I thought they would be safe, that all the foreign funds in the purse had been stolen. I recalled when a huge amount of funds was stolen from me in my own home; the money just disappeared from where I kept it. I remembered the time a couple of persons charged with the responsibility of helping us with our building project had cheated us and we lost a lot of money in the process. I realised that the pain and hurt of being deprived of things belonging to me was still festering in the deep crevices of my heart. The more I pondered on it, the more I realised that I had to pray and release the hurt into the hands of God. I asked the Lord to help me to forgive and let it go. I received the grace to forgive all these people. They cannot pay me back what they have taken from me but the Lord promised that He will abundantly repay.

It was already eighteen months at that time that I could not work as a result of the chronic infirmity. I considered that if I had been working here in Geneva as a local staff at the time when I became too ill to continue to work and had to stop working on health grounds, I would have qualified to receive disability allowance. Each time I visited the hospital for respiratory rehabilitation, the social workers asked me if I was receiving disability allowance and I had to respond that I was not qualified because I had separated on medical grounds after working for twelve years of active continuous service but as a contract staff. I could not renew my contract because of the state of my health so I was not able to receive any allowance from my organisation as well. I had no grounds on which to claim disability allowance or compensation for not being able to work because of my health.

> The pain we feel in the waiting season may cloud the hope we have. Therein lies the challenge; this is when we must consciously and with strong determination keep our focus on our expectation and the object.

The ability to work was stolen from me. The opportunity to work was stolen from me. Because of the infirmity I could not apply for jobs that I was professionally qualified for. The compensation for not being able to work was stolen from me. So much of my time and energy was consumed every day as I spent valuable time managing the affliction, doing all the essential routines of dealing and coping with the disease. I reckoned that my time is a very valuable resource but not only mine but that of my husband, my children and every person who has had to care for me without pay. Yet, all of these were stolen by the enemy of my soul.

The Bible says in Proverbs 6:31 that when a thief is caught, he must repay seven times what he had stolen even if it he has to sell everything in his house to repay. I also know the devil comes to steal, to kill and to destroy. I recognise who the thief is; it is the devil. I cannot even begin to enumerate all the things that I know he stole from me through the course of this infirmity, not to talk of the ones that I do not even know about. The ones I enumerated above were just a tip of the iceberg. What about all our resources that went into the daily medications I have to consume, the hospital bills, medical equipment and services. Need I mention the boxes of tissues or packs of convenience towels consumed over the years? These are the many ways the devil had stolen and wasted our resources. Based on the word of God, I have a solid argument to claim a compensation. There has to be a payback time. The thief must repay. But this thief cannot pay me back. He cannot repay what he has stolen from me.

Ruminating on this almost tipped me into a phase of anger as sorrow welled up in my heart. That was when I read Genesis

15:1, as God spoke to Abram, "I am your Shield, your abundant compensation and exceedingly great reward." I felt the Holy Spirit illuminating the word of God in my heart in a brand new way that brought me hope and comfort. Only God is able to abundantly compensate my family and me for all that we lost, all that I have been deprived off, and all that has been destroyed and devoured from my life. I claim double for my many troubles. I stand on the authority of the Word that all my years that the woodworm, the palmerworm and caterpillar have consumed shall be restored to me in Jesus name. God promised that I will recover without fail all that the enemy had stolen from me, and with recompense. I chose to stand on God's promise.

God says, "He is my abundant compensation and exceedingly great reward". He will pay me back abundantly, He will give me recompense and He will cause the retroactive to be given to me in Jesus name. I can lay claim on the restoration, the recompense, the retroactive and the payback, standing on the authority of God's infallible promise and in the name of Jesus. I can begin to give thanks to God for the recompense and reward. God is able to cause the book of remembrance to be opened on my behalf. He can bring to remembrance all that is due me that I have been deprived off and have it given to me retroactively. He is able to do the never done before, the never heard of before for my sake to ensure that I am abundantly compensated for all that I have lost as a result of this affliction. This message of hope and reassurance would become even the more important as the story of my life unfolds and I enter into the season of recovery.

There was no longer any point for me to waste my energy pursuing anyone to payback what they owe me, or what they have stolen from me. They cannot pay me back. I will look unto

God, who is faithful and who is just to bring justice into my life and give me recompense. After all, those who put their trust in the Him will never be ashamed. My expectation is not of man but it is of God. I am expecting from the Lord and when the Lord gives, He gives abundantly. He is able to do exceedingly, super-abundantly more that I could ever dream, think, imagine, desire or even dare to ask. Way beyond my expectation, God is able to provide and compensate me because He Himself is my compensation. So I began to dream big and have a head-size expectation, being persuaded that I will surely testify of it as it comes to pass because Faithful is He who has promised.

2009 ended on a beautiful note, with me full of praise and thanks for God's love and superabundant mercies towards me and my family. Despite the many odds, we made it into the new year joyfully.

#

Living Today Waiting For A Miracle

It was April 2010. It was the time for life to resurrect from the dead—a season of newness and freshness. The earth begins reawakening in earnest announcing that Spring has arrived. This was supposed to be the season of refreshing and renewal after the long winter. Brilliant yellow canola set to spring out of the fallow grounds. The green leaves had started sprouting on the trees outside my bedroom window—transforming the dry twiggy trees to a luscious green. But I felt no transformation or refreshing in my body. It had been another rough and long night. I sat at my usual place at the edge of my bed staring out through the window at the blue sky with only a few scattered grey clouds.

"How long, O Lord? How long before my miracle will come?" I cried out in silence. "How do I live each day waiting for my miracle?" I dragged myself up from the bed and went into the room opposite mine, turned on the computer. I needed to write a letter to God or perhaps to a few men of faith in the Bible who had waited for long for the promise to be fulfilled and for their miracle to come. There are questions I would love to ask them. Maybe their answers will help me get through this drawn out winter season of my life. That was how I wrote my letter to some of the heroes of our faith:

"There are a few persons I wish I could sit down and talk to today. I would like to find out how they lived day to day waiting for a miracle; waiting for the fulfilment of the promise they hold true and dear to heart. I would love to ask them a few questions about how they dealt with the pain they felt or the enormity of their circumstances which ran contrary to the hope they were clinging to.

First on my list is Father Abraham, he knew Sarah was barren when God first promised him He would make him a great nation. How did he get up each morning and face each passing day while he watched his wife advance in years until she was passed the age of child bearing?

Yes, I do know that he believed that God, who has the divine power to give life to the dead and to call those things which are not as if they already existed, is able to quicken his aged body and the dead womb of Sarah. He held on to that without wavering. The promise was not fulfilled in one year or ten years, he waited for a long time to see Isaac born. What was going through his mind during those long years of waiting? How was he living each day and how did he encourage Sarah to hold on to the promise?

Next, I would love to sit and chat with Sarah, called the mother of nations but bore daily the enormous burden of barrenness. Each passing month brought her closer to the end of the road as far as it was humanly possible for her to have a child. What was the state of her mind when she asked her husband to sleep with her servant? How did she handle the pain and agony of the contempt Hagar showed towards her? I can imagine how ridiculous it must have sounded being told at 90 years of age that she was going to have a child after all. No wonder she laughed. I would like to ask her how she felt the following morning looking at her body.

I sat there until it got to the point that I knew I had to call my soul to order and switch off the channel I was watching in my head. That was when I began to pour out my heart to God.

I closed my eyes and imagined her putting her hand over her stomach and wondering if it was truly going to protrude, wondering what she would look like pregnant. Every woman who has waited on the Lord for a child would understand what I am talking about. Standing in front of a mirror, touching the abdomen and trying to imagine what it would look like carrying a child. Surely Sarah must have done that too.

Certainly today, I feel like talking with Hannah harassed by Penninah who mocked her childlessness and relentlessly provoked her sore. What was it like for her waking up each day to the cry of Penninah's children and their laughter as they ran around playing? What was going on in her mind when she approached the altar and broke down in a fervent silent prayer that made her look like one who had consumed too much alcohol and in a drunken state? The Bible recorded that she cried no more after she received the promise of a child. But did that promise stop her from wondering when the promise would be fulfilled?

"Talk to me, you great men and women who know what it means to wait and wait and wait?" Tears welled up and streamed down my cheeks. "My heart is in great distress. Talk to me."

Definitely, I want to have a chat with the woman with the issue of blood. The Bible did not record her name. I would particularly love to listen to her share her testimony of how she lived for twelve years with an intractable problem that seemed like it would never go away. Because that is how I feel right now, I have been coughing for seventeen years and I can relate to this woman. I had the opportunity to study her story and to place it in contemporary times five years ago when it was also twelve years with this affliction I face. As a nutrition scientist, I could put one of the fallouts of her problem in context; chronic anaemia and all that goes with it including weakness, lethargia etc. I imagined the issues of hygiene she would have had to deal with at a time when facilities for such would have been limited.

How did she cope with such a seemingly hopeless situation on a day-to-day basis? Where did she find the strength to push against the throng of people surrounding Jesus until she got close enough to touch the hem of His garment?

Of course, I really must talk with Brother Paul. He bore in his flesh a thorn. What that thorn was, we know not. But this one thing we do know, he did not want it! He wished he did not have it and he pleaded with God three times to take it away from him. We know that the thorn buffeted him, assailed him and harassed him, may be even humiliated him. It must have distressed him and possibly caused him a lot of pain. But in it, Paul received the grace to remain strong and be encouraged; the grace to go through without complaining.

Today, I feel buffeted and harassed. The distress and pain is simply too much to bear and I long so much for instant relief. Even though I could not sit physically with these dear witnesses, I feel their comfort coming through as I write this message; meditating again on their lives. I can see the wonderful works of God in

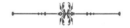

This verse tells me that God has the power to break the yoke of self-pity and to deliver from despair and depression. When we worship and praise God, when we give Him a sacrifice of thanksgiving, burdens are lifted, yokes are broken and the restraining bars of iron are cut asunder.

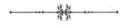

them. They have been where I am now. They seem to be gathered all around me right now as they comfort me with the same comfort with which they have been comforted. Yes, I feel the same grace that abounded to them flowing towards me to lift up my head and hold me up."

As I recalled the deeds of the Lord and called to remembrance His wonderful miracles of old, His peace flooded my heart. So I purposed in my heart that I will turn my mind to meditate upon all His works and consider all His mighty hands have done as I live today, waiting for my miracle. I will not stop thinking about them but will ponder on them and ensure that they are constantly in my thoughts to drive away all doubts. My meditation will be on the greatness of the Lord and the power He has demonstrated on behalf of His people, and that will lift up my heart and spirit in confidence that God who did not spare His Only Son but delivered Him up to die a cruel death for me, will with Jesus freely give me all things. Indeed, that power that raised Christ from the dead and gave Him victory over the grave is at work in me and on my behalf right now.

Praise welled up in my heart and I began to shout "Hallelujah, all praise and thanks be to God."

I decided to face each day with renewed confidence and trust in God. I received for each day an unusual measure of trust to believe in God's given ability to do the miraculous for me in this seemly impossible situation. I am persuaded that He who keeps covenant with day and night is faithful, reliable and true to His word. For as long as day follows after night, I know that He would do what He says He would do concerning me. I receive with thanksgiving the measure of grace and strength to go through each day standing steadfast on His sure promises.

#

Never Give Up On Hope

I give thanks to God Who never leaves His own desolate or alone. It is uplifting and such a blessing to know that we have a God who will never leave any of His children desolate in the midst of the storm or in times of adversity and hardship. Desolate, in the sense that one feels abandoned and devoid of help, hope and comfort. I give thanks to God for His unfailing and compassionate love for me. The reassurance of His love often shines out to me like a beam of light through dark clouds.

My health had been on such a roller-coaster that sometimes I felt like crawling into a corner and crying. And there were times I just gave in to my emotions and wept. My husband told me repeatedly that we don't have to be religious with God. We can tell Him how we feel and He will respond to us in the way that

My husband kept encouraging me. He recounted the word of God to me.

will best minister to us. This reminded me of Job's sincerity when he poured out his heart out to God, undiluted and unfiltered. I marvelled at how God responded to him such that at the end of it all, Job had to acknowledge that no one else can deliver or fight for us but God.

In the trial of my faith, sometimes I wanted my miracle to be instant, at that very second. There were times I got tired of being constantly tired. I got tired of being too fatigued to do the things I love doing. There were many times I felt constrained and limited, when it seemed that I could not bear the pain and distress one minute longer. At moments, such as described, I thank God because He came through for me. He sent His word and it bound my wounds, both physical and emotional.

I was at one of such moments in October 2010. Over the past years, I committed myself to doing something different during my birth-month to enhance my walk and deepen my relationship with the Lord. This time I decided to do a partial fast. The drugs I take and the effect of the drugs on my tummy had made it difficult for me to abstain from eating. I also decided to study the "Never Give Up! Curriculum" by Joyce Meyer. It was an apt subject for me to study at that time. I read the book. I did the Bible study. I learnt as much as I could on what the Bible had to say about hope. I wanted to know everything there is to know about hope. So I searched the dictionary. I liked the definition that hope is an optimistic attitude of mind based on an expectation of positive outcomes related to events and circumstances in one's life. It is a strong and confident expectation.

> **I knew I had to deal with the anger immediately. Otherwise, not only would the seed of offense take root in my heart but also the feeling of despair will engulf me.**

There was included in the package a teal coloured bracelet with Never Give Up inscribed boldly in black. I wore this bracelet every day for almost three years, until the day I was wheeled into the theatre in April 2013. I added my own inscription on the bracelet based on what I had learnt during the extensive Bible Study. These were words that I wanted to keep in view and constantly remember:

> I am relentless
> I am adamant
> I am unyielding

These are attributes of hope. Hope must be relentless and steadfast in pursuit of seeing what it is expecting. I knew I could not afford to give up on hope. Indeed, for me to lose hope is to give up on life. I was once close to that in 2008 but for the mercy of God, I would not have lived to tell the story.

I must stubbornly hold on to the hope of living a full healthy life again. I must be relentless in pursuit of my dreams and expectation of the Lord. I must be unyielding in my expectation that I will live to see the goodness of the Lord in the land of the living.

> **Praise lifted me out of the pit and refocused my attention on the unfailing love of God for me.**

"For in hope we have been saved...if we hope for what we do not see, with perseverance we wait eagerly for it." (Romans 8:24-25)

This hymn composed by Segtimus Winner in 1868 whispered hope to my heart;

> *Soft as the voice of an angel,*
> *Breathing a lesson unheard,*
> *Hope with a gentle persuasion*
> *Whispers her comforting word:*
> *Wait till the darkness is over,*
> *Wait till the tempest is done,*
> *Hope for the sunshine tomorrow,*
> *After the shower is gone.*
> *Refrain:*
> *Whispering hope, oh, how welcome thy voice,*
> *Making my heart in its sorrow rejoice.*

Hope does not make us ashamed. It does not disappoint. Because the love of God is poured out generously into our hearts and we know how much He loves us, He asked His Holy Spirit to fill our hearts with His love (Romans 5:5). It is this assurance of the love that God has so generously poured into our hearts that provides a solid rock for hope to anchor on.

Giving thanks in all circumstances then becomes something you consciously order your soul to do.

The pain we feel in the waiting season may cloud the hope we have. Therein lies the challenge; this is when we must consciously and with strong determination keep our focus on our expectation and the object. It is when we must choose never to give up, come what may. It is a choice but there is grace available to enable and empower us.

#

The Reproach of Affliction

Lisa was leaving Switzerland at the end of the week. Her husband's tour of service in the country had ended and they were relocating to the United States before their next posting. Lisa and I had spent many hours in prayers along with our sisters in the Mum's prayer group—praying for our children, their school and our husbands for over two years. All the other Mums had left on summer vacation. Lisa was packing. I could not travel with my husband and sons on university visit in the United States because I had been grounded by my doctors.

It was our last afternoon together. We recalled the many prayers we had raised up to God during our time together over lunch in a Chinese restaurant on Route de Suisse. We offered praises to God for the many answers to our prayers and for His awesome work in the lives of our children and husbands. Lisa had been such a tremendous blessing to me and my family in so many ways. Beyond praying, she was a true friend and a help indeed - cooked many dinners for us and drove me to places I needed to be. I was going to miss her greatly.

We finished lunch, lingered a bit more chatting and it was time to leave. The hostess opened the door to let us out and as we stepped outside, hot air so thick that you could cut with a knife enveloped me. It had been a hot humid summer in 2010 but that afternoon, the sauna hot humid heat was made it difficult for me to breathe. My head was swimming by the time I crossed the short distance between the door and the car.

"Are you alright?" Lisa asked, looking alarmed.

"I can't breathe," I whispered. I had switched to the second oxygen bottle in the restaurant. I knew my oxygen saturation had dropped. I needed more oxygen. She helped me to the car. I increased the oxygen flow and started taking deep breaths. But it was as if the air was too thick to go down.

"Should I call the ambulance?"

I shook my head vigorously. I didn't want the ambulance. The people coming out of the restaurant were standing around. The heat was making it difficult to breathe. It was even hotter inside the car than outside. I knew I had to get oxygen down into my lungs fast. And that was went it happened. The amount of oxygen in my blood had become so low and I felt my muscles becoming slack. I lost control of my sphincter muscles and my bladder emptied right there on the car seat. The shame and embarrassment that stung my face with heat was hotter than the heat of the sun blazing overhead. Tears welled up as I covered my face in shame. "Not again, not again." I sobbed in the depth of my soul but not a sound escaped from my lips though the groans were loud within.

> **I had to, at this dark moment of my life, find my worth defined in who He called me to be.**

> **The more I found reasons to be grateful, the more thanks I expressed, the more my spirit was lifted up, and the more joy overflowed in my heart.**

After what seemed like forever, I composed myself and summoned the courage to lift my head up. I had to tell Lisa what had happened. She was planning to take the car for cleaning that afternoon before putting it up for sale. She needed to know and would find out anyway.

"We can go now." I mumbled, looking up to her. She had been standing covering me from passers-by with one arm on the door and the other on top the car. Her body blocked the sun rays from me. My head became stable and stopped swimming. Oxygen saturation had improved but my heart was heavy. I was grieved and in pain in the depth of my soul.

"There's something I need to tell you, Lisa." She was behind the steering, ready to drive out of the park. She paused and turned towards me; I began to narrate my story. She was very understanding and kept assuring me that it was alright. I couldn't stop apologising all the way back home. I offered to clean up the car but she wouldn't hear of it. Her empathy gave me the grace to step out of the car without covering my face when we got to my house. Experience in the past had taught me to always have a shawl handy in the few times that I go out, so that I will have something to wrap myself with in the event of an accident such as this. But this was the worst of it all. Lisa got out of the car and came around to my side. She gave me a huge hug that was so comforting and reassuring; yet the pain in my heart was unassuaged. Grieved to the core of my being that a very lovely afternoon and the time we shared together ended on such a painfully embarrassing note.

> It requires looking at our circumstance and yet focusing on the truth of who God is irrespective of what we may be going through.

I went straight to my room and into the bathroom to strip off the wet cloths. Cleaned up, I sat in bed with my arms wrapped around my knees drawn up against my chin. I began to play the movie of the years I had lived with the shame of urinary incontinence exacerbated by the chronic respiratory disease. These incessant bouts of coughing had provoked me beyond words. I was at the rock bottom, totally numb. My husband was thousands of kilometres away and there was no one I could share my pain with or pour out my heart to.

It started in 1999; the frequent bouts of coughing began to put too much pressure on my bladder to the extent that I had to empty my bladder as frequent as possible to prevent leakage during coughing. But the more I coughed the drier my throat became and the more water I wanted to drink to sooth my throat. This meant frequent trips to the bathroom. The situation became more difficult to handle when traveling. Since my job was 40% travel, it soon became obvious that I had another problem to deal with on top of the respiratory and neuro-muscular diseases. We couldn't just stop anywhere for me to use the bathroom. It became increasingly difficult to hold my bladder. So I started drinking less before and during trips, and used more menthol sweets to sooth my throat. But it did not always work out well.

I remembered the day I arrived at the Delta State Government House for an advocacy meeting with the State Governor. I coughed all the way 150 kilometres from Benin City, where we spent the previous night, to Asaba, the capital city of Delta State. I felt the wetness and knew that disaster was in the making again. I instinctively swung my shawl over my hips as I got out of the white UNICEF Land cruiser, and headed straight for the bathroom as soon as we were received into the Government House. I had learnt never to leave the vehicle without checking my skirt. Low and behold, the leak had caused a wet blot on my olive coloured short tailored skirt. Thankfully, there was a hair dryer in the bathroom. Even more thankful that I was alone throughout the time I needed to dry my skirt. That was the last time I wore a light coloured skirt suit for an official engagement outside the office. I changed my work wardrobe to pant suits, which were easier to manage and my jackets were long enough to cover my hips. I chose dark colours that will not easily reveal accidental wetness. There were no convenience towels in those days. Sanitary towels simply could not hold the heavy leaks.

I blessed God for the day my husband and I finally found convenience towels in a shop in Geneva. We stockpiled them. I had a bag full of the towels when I left for Cairo to return back to work. I restocked each time I went back to Geneva at the end of each month. My muscles were frequently becoming slack during episodes of oxygen insufficiency. Cairo was particularly challenging with the heat and dust, which worsened my respiratory situation to the extent that I became oxygen-dependent. I started having more frequent episodes of oxygen insufficiency. Soon the towels started giving way with the increasing volume of leaks especially during travels. I carried several packs in my bag and a trash bag as well, always looking for opportunities to empty my bladder and check to be sure that I was containing the leaks.

Several embarrassing episodes later, I returned back to Geneva. I stopped working. I went out of the house only when necessary and mostly on Sundays to church. Inspite of my best efforts to manage the problem, which I did not even have the courage to discuss with my doctors, there were still episodes of wet blots on my dress and on the car seat especially after a severe bout of coughing. It was just too shameful to talk about it. And honestly, I did not want to add one more condition on the list of the complex multi-systemic afflictions my doctors were trying to manage.

One day, I got fed-up with the whole thing that I summoned the courage to discuss with a doctor who was standing in for my regular doctor. But before she could have it fully investigated, my respiratory problem got out of hand again and urinary incontinence fell off the chart.

Each episode I replayed in my mind on that fateful summer afternoon drove the knife of grief deeper and deeper into the core of my being. I felt the pain of Hannah provoked sore by Peninnah combined with the shame of the woman with the issue of blood for twelve years. It was as if all the different issues had connived to shame, embarrass and taunt me. That was the day Psalm 34:19 took a new meaning for me.

A significant amount of human communication takes place, not in words, but in gestures.

"Many are the afflictions of the righteous, But the LORD delivers him out of them all."

I sat there until it got to the point that I knew I had to call my soul to order and switch off the channel I was watching in my head. That was when I began to pour out my heart to God. I pleaded my case before the throne of grace. It took a long while before the 'BUT' sank in, before I took note of what came after the BUT—the Lord delivers him out of them ALL. The Lord delivers me out of all these many afflictions. That is the promise of God. I allowed this word to sink to the depth of my soul where the heat of hurt was burning the most. God promised that instead of shame, He will give me double portion. He also promised that I would not be put to shame and He will remove reproach from me.

I cried louder to God to remove from me the reproach and the shame of these afflictions. I didn't know how much longer it would take but I was persuaded that God will not renege on any of these promises. If He said He will remove the reproach of these afflictions, He will surely do so in His own time and in His own way. I knew I had to release the pain and grief in my heart and allowed myself to be comforted with God's promise and the grace with which Lisa had handled the situation. For that I was extremely thankful. I was thankful that she did not add to my reproach. The way she held me and hugged me echoed God's love for me. If Lisa who had every logical reason to be ashamed of me could hold me and hug me, I knew the King of kings who is the gracious God is not ashamed of me. I felt Him drawing me into the hollow of His comforting arms, and He lifted me out of that pit of reproach, despair and shame

#

Praise That Breaks The Yoke

"O that men will praise the Lord, for His goodness, and for His wonderful works to the children of men! He has broken the gates of brass and cut the bars of iron in asunder." – Ps 107:15-16.

I found myself singing a song based on this verse during the week of November 16, 2011. I paused to ponder on the verse. Brass and iron are hard metals, which is why you can make gates and bars with them including prison gates, shackles and bars. The verse revealed to me the infinite and mighty power of God to deal with hard and knotty issues in our lives, and the complex situations we often have to face. Difficult times in our lives can drive us to self-pity, despair and sometimes depression. Many people who have experienced knotty and complex situations can testify of the feeling of heaviness and a sense of hopelessness that can accompany despair, which in itself holds the individual bound as with a heavy shackle or yoke.

That was the birth of my blog captioned "Enriching Lives, Inspiring Hope". The address was TouchingLives4good-- that is what we prayed that each blog post would do; enrich lives, inspire hope and touch lives for good.

This verse tells me that God has the power to break the yoke of self-pity and to deliver from despair and depression. When we worship and praise God, when we give Him a sacrifice of thanksgiving, burdens are lifted, yokes are broken and the restraining bars of iron are cut asunder. Let me share my experience in this regard.

Towards the end of 2010, my doctors suggested to me the option of having a surgical procedure, which they deemed the only medical option left to address the progressively worsening respiratory difficulties I was experiencing. I remembered my husband and I were sitting in my doctor's office when he proposed to us that the only option left for me to have a chance at living a full life was to have lung transplantation. I was speechless. It was as if I was hearing Prof. PJ talking from a long distance as he explained the investigations he had made to provide justifications for me to be considered for transplantation. His voice was faint. My mind had travelled far away from the room. I stared over his shoulders through the window behind him into the blue sky overhead. As faint as his voice was, it was distinct; I did not miss a word he said.

"Whose report would you believe?" my husband asked as we walked on the mustard yellow tiles down the long corridor away from Prof. PJ's office. "We will believe the report of the Lord" I responded. It was like a dream. I wanted to wake up quickly from the dream but it held fast to me. I could not get my head around the thought of having lung transplantation. I knew what was required to happen for me to get a set of lungs. My imagination went riot and I did not know how to pray. How could I possibly ask God to give someone for me? That's what I would be asking for if I prayed about this - for God to find me a new set of lungs someone would have to pay the ultimate price. I could not allow my mind to contemplate that thought so I simply put it out of my mind - at least for a season.

Prof. PJ, having made a solid case for me to be considered for transplantation transferred my case to the Transplantation Team of the hospital. That was when I met Dr. PSG. I did not know what to make of her at the beginning. I had become accustomed to Prof. PJ and the way he had hitherto managed my case. We had built a relationship over the years. My husband and I had grown to respect him and his opinion. He assured me that he would still be closely associated with me but Dr PSG will be taking the lead from that point. I knew we were entering another season. I would have to learn to build a relationship with my new doctor. I prayed that she would always act in my best interest as Prof. PJ had, and beyond my medical history, I desired that she would relate with me as a person not as a case. This was very important to me.

Because of the risks associated with this procedure I was required to have a full medical workup to ensure that I qualified for the transplantation and to ensure that the other medical problems I had would not pose additional risks to me both during and after the surgery. I had to go to another hospital which was the designated centre for lungs transplantation for my region. It was located some 60 kilometres away from Geneva in another city, Lausanne. During the medical workup, I met with all the specialists who were likely to be involved in the procedure. Afterward, I got a preliminary clearance for the procedure. But one of the surgeons was very concerned about my medical history, which he deemed complex and he felt that this would not only pose additional risk to the surgery but that it was a sufficient reason not to do it at all. He wanted to review the case again more thoroughly before agreeing to the procedure. He was the head of the surgical team in charge of lung transplantation and a senior professor. The Old Prophet as I would refer to him in this book was so brusque in presenting the facts that his words fell like a heavy load of bricks on me. I felt suffocated listening to him. I tried hard to shake the weight of his words off but they weighed heavy on my spirit.

When we left his office to wait to see the other specialists, my husband kept encouraging me. He recounted the word of God to me. It was not the first time that we had left a doctor's office and we had to confess that we know whose report we would believe. We believe in the report of the Lord and His report says "I am healed." Although all the other specialists we saw were optimistic about the procedure, the report of the Old prophet pinned me down. We talked about what happened all the way from Lausanne back to Geneva with my husband simply doing his best to take my mind off the verdict of the Old Prophet and keep my focus on the promise of God, as he drove on the AutoRoute. My vision was blurred. I stared out through the window but saw nothing. My mind was too muddled. I was seething with anger and resentment. I could not keep my focus on the word of God my husband was sharing with me.

I went straight to my bedroom as soon as we got home and began to wail before God. I was very angry with the Old Prophet and I resented the offhanded way he addressed the issue. While I agreed he had the responsibility to present all the facts I felt he could have done so without making the situation look so hopeless. I felt overwhelmed by the heaviness in my spirit. All I could do was wail from the depth of my heart. I knew I had to deal with the anger immediately. Otherwise, not only would the seed of offense take root in my heart but also the feeling of despair will engulf me. I slept off that night out of sheer exhaustion.

> Yet it was at one of such times as these that I was reminded to endure with joy and maintain a joyful attitude.

The following morning, I told my husband I was not coming out of the room until I could open my mouth and give praise to God. I asked him to set up the iPod to play some praise and worship songs to help lift my spirit. After listening to the songs for a while, I found myself meditating on the lyrics and soon I was singing along, first quietly and then loudly. Don Moen's song "I will sing" particularly ministered to me. As I sang; "I will sing, I will praise even in my darkest hour ... Lift my hands to honour You because Your word is true, I will sing" over and over again, the flood gate busted open, and tears began to flow uncontrolled. At first, I was wailing out of pain and out of the vexation of my heart. But it changed as I sang and wept. It was no longer a wail of despair but the tears were flowing from an overwhelming assurance of God's love for me. I felt His arms holding me in His bosom and His breath breathed peace that enveloped my heart. A confident hope was rekindled in me that He would not allow me to be tried more than I could bear. The more I sang praise, the lighter my spirit became. The power of that praise kept me from the brink of self-pity and despair.

The pressured times in our lives are like the processing that every raw material must go through so that a great and high quality product can be made of out them.

I knew then that praise and adoration of God has the power to break the iron bars of grief and despair and the brass gates of hopelessness. When circumstances in our lives push us to the brink of despair, praise holds us from falling over the precipice. Praise breaks the yoke of self-pity, despair and depression. If I entertained the anger, offense and self-pity, I would have been given to that destructive emotion of despair, which would have drained me of hope and strength. But taking on praise kept me in check. Praise lifted me out of the pit and refocused my attention on the unfailing love of God for me.

#

Gratitude in the Caves of Confinement

Giving thanks when everything is good and rosy is not difficult at all; the challenge in giving thanks and exhibiting a grateful attitude is when things are not going your way, when things are out of your control and when the things you desire seem to be out of your reach. Giving thanks in all circumstances then becomes something you consciously order your soul to do.

In the course of the week leading to December 14th, 2011, I came to appreciate better what it must have been like for Jesus to be despised. The Son of God hanging on the cross with all the shame of iniquity and many afflictions laid upon Him. Separated from His glory just because of me—held guilty and literally punished for the sin He did not commit.

When you are treated as if guilty of an offense and yet you don't know what your crime is. When you know you are also a victim but that does not seem to matter. At such moments, it takes more than will power not to shout out--why me? What have I done to deserve this? What have I neglected to do to prevent this? What do you do when the label of your affliction screamed like a bill board and the restraints of isolation felt like hangman's noose choking life out of you? Imagine for a moment a day in the life of the woman with the issue of blood who suffered many things in the hands of the physicians. When your affliction becomes the label by which people identify and treat you, it hurts and deeply too. Every muscle fibre in you seems to cry out--this is not fair! I was at that point during my stay at the Respiratory Rehabilitation Hospital in a town about 25 km from Geneva in December 2011.

Room 217 at the end of the corridor became a place of isolation. The brilliant yellow frames that once enhanced the mellow maize hues of the walls of the room became its label to containment. Nothing left the room except bagged in yellow plastic bags. A yellow flag posted on the door signalled, "Keep off" to many. Only the essential staff entered the room. The room where dreams were once freely conceived now imposed severe restraints. The nurses' cherry faces that once beamed smiles at me were now hid behind green masks above which their eyes peeked at me, some with pity and some as if beholding someone with a plague. Their hands that once freely touched me concealed in gloves were cold. They no longer lingered for a chat. It was as if they could not wait to be out of the room. Some did not like the rules of the quarantine but they were compelled to comply. These ones wanted me to keep smiling as usual and take it in my stride. Others from a significant distance dished out their instructions. I was grieved to the very core of my being. Within these four walls I was confined twenty-three hours a day for sixteen days with one hour away to the gruelling press of the Physiotherapy gym. I longed for this precious one hour away from my cave of confinement. Though I was required to be covered in green overall with face mask and gloves on, it was still an escape. I could see other faces, hear their voices and watch them struggling at their own press. But the hour always passed quickly. At the beginning, I fidgeted, groaned and complained--loudly too.

> I could not have survived the ordeal without the hope that only Jesus gives.

Knowing God always has a purpose and a reason for every experience He permits me to go through did not offer much comfort at that point in time. All I saw were the barriers and how restraining they were. I focused on them until those yellow walls loomed like the high walls of a maximum-security prison.

I took a long look at the stranger in the mirror and I began to speak the Word of God, the word of life to her.

It was at that low ebb that the song by Tommy Walker filtered into my spirit;

"When I don't know what to do, I'll lift my hands, when I don't know what to say, I'll speak Your praise."

It commanded me to be a worshipper. I searched for the song and sang it over and over again. Along with it also came; "Grateful, Lord I am grateful for all You've done for me" by Kurt Carr. These two songs became my close companions and source of comfort in that dark valley. I knew that gratitude of necessity must be my attitude even in all that was going through. I must admit that it was with reluctance that I yielded. Yes, I was grateful for all God had done for me. But it was with the deep pain and hurt in my heart, that I expressed my gratitude to God; "Even though You slay me, yet I will still praise You." I was grateful God was with me. I was grateful for His comfort. He lifted up my head and kept it held high. I had to, at this dark moment of my life, find my worth defined in who He called me to be. At such times as I was in, it is so important for us to know who we are in Christ Jesus, and to hinge our worth on Him. No matter how hard the devil tries he cannot redefine who we are in Christ Jesus, if we don't let him.

Gratitude and joy are intricately woven together. The more I found reasons to be grateful, the more thanks I expressed, the more my spirit was lifted up, and the more joy overflowed in my heart. So I chose to stay on the path of gratitude--took a look back into the year and began to count the many things I had to be grateful for. I was grateful for the new friends made, new contacts established, divinely engineered connections, many new beginnings... My list became quite long in the process. I considered also the many "what ifs"—the alternate possibilities that God delivered us from. A stretch of imagination alone will cause us to be grateful for the unseen Hands of God working on our behalf and for His faithfulness to His word.

We all have our different stories of the sufferings and difficulties we have to endure - some physical, some emotional. When we endure the heat of the trials, a beautiful and godly character is produced in us as precious metals are refined in fire (1Peter 1:6-7). God will never allow us to be tried beyond what we can bear but with every trial He makes a way for escape (1Corinthians 10:13). The way of escape for me was to switch my focus from the pain and distress to the many blessings God has poured into my life. With that came the lightening of the burden--it took the sting out of the pain - it prepared me to receive the comfort only God could give.

Whatever struggles we may be faced with, God will always provide a way of escape. One ready way is to have an attitude of gratitude and to give thanks even in that situation. It requires looking at our circumstance and yet focusing on the truth of who God is irrespective of what we may be going through.

"Gratitude is born in hearts that take time to count past mercies." - Charles E. Jefferson

Beauty In The Cave

Pressed against the hard rock
Under immerse pressure
In the midst of trials
Often when most discomforted
An idea, brilliant and germane, is
conceived
A character, tried and true, is birthed
A gem, beautiful to behold, is produced
In the furnace of affliction
The promises of God shine brightly

The waiting room, the place where the Word becomes to you a life line.

As gratitude permeated the atmosphere of my cave of confinement, I began to take notice of small details within room 217. I noticed how brilliant the hues on the drapes were set against the darkness of the night and how the colours seemed to fade when sunlight filtered through them. I noticed every colour and detail of the pattern on the walls, on the floor and wood of the table -- changing with the light of day and night, and I knew God does not change.

One night, distressed with the choking, head resting on my hands, elbows burrowed into my laps, I sat on my bed and declared, "Thank You God, thank You because I have hope, thank You that I know Your promises concerning me."

In close proximity and quietness, I paid attention to the things I would have missed in the hurried busyness of life. Through the windows, I saw sun rays glow against the snow-capped mountains in a kaleidoscope of fiery orange upon the grey clouds scattered in the blue sky. Lake Leman appeared aquamarine as the setting sun cast a golden beam upon it. The next day, it turned opaque under a heavy cloak of fog and its surroundings draped with a blanket of snow. Reflecting on the beauty of His nature—changing through the season—I knew God remains unchanging.

In the long hours of solitude, the voice of God filtered clearly through my often cluttered mind nudging me to give thanks in all things and at all times. At the time when it almost seemed too hard to go on, I heard "I am with you." He gave me many assurances of His abiding presence and He encouraged my faith. He sharpened my focus and tuned my ears to listen. I learnt of Him in a new way confined within the wall of room 217.

You can make your time in the waiting room worthwhile by being busy doing good.

"I can do all things through Christ Who strengthens me" became my watch word at the press. There is a purpose for this test and a reason for this trial. There is something He is preparing me for and I needed to go through this period to be ready for it. God gives the strength and the grace to overcome and to gain victory.

I will forever be grateful to God for His faithfulness and for His love. Now I can say I am truly grateful for the experience of Room 217 at the end of the corridor and for all God used that experience to birth in me. Pressed against the hard rock, my muscles toned up and became stronger. Strength and stamina returned with every effort made to endure the extra mile. Against the hard rock, His grace abounded and His promises became sure. I emerged from room 217 knowing a brand new thread had been woven by God's mighty hands into the tapestry He is weaving of my life. Another piece was added to the puzzle of the picture He has in mind of me. With this in mind, I always will cherish the times spent in Room 217. I will nurture the dreams conceived in the room. But it has fulfilled its mission. I never again want to be within those four walls.

Be assured that in the midst of your trial and testing, God is making a gem beautiful to behold out of you if you hold on.

"We are hard pressed on every side, but not crushed; perplexed, but not in despair" – 2Corinthians 4:8(NIV)

When we rode out of the Rehabilitation Hospital just three days to Christmas, I purposed in my heart that it was the last time I would be in that hospital. I was not going back to that cave of confinement and isolation anymore. I knew I was required to have the annual rehabilitation to improve my respiratory status. But for as long as the plague of pseudomonas will condemn me to isolation, I felt I could not maximally benefit from the program. Secondly, the psychological impact of the isolation was tremendous. My doctors also understood this, because at a point, they called in a psychiatrist to evaluate my mental health. Though my anger, for a while, was directed at the medical and nursing team, I understood that they were simply doing what is required by hospital regulations to prevent the spread of the infection to other patients. They had to act in the best interest of the other patients. What was difficult for me to appreciate was that for most of them the requirements of the "law" was implemented without a human face. I was not the plague. I am a human being with feelings and emotions. When a nurse refused to touch a cup that I touched or stood at a distance to give me information while telling me she could not come closer because she was not wearing the protective clothing and she held the face mask to her face with her hand, it conveyed a far-reaching message of insensitivity.

I could relate at that point with the lepers in the Biblical times that were isolated from families and friends because the Jewish regulations prohibited contact with other people to prevent the spread of the disease. How lonely and isolated they must have felt prohibited from human touch for so many years. You can then imagine the joy of the leper in Luke Chapter 5, when Jesus stretched out His hands and touched the leper. He reached out and touched the man with leprosy, the man who had been prohibited from being touched, who had no physical touch for many years, isolated from his family and friends. A significant amount of human communication takes place, not in words, but in gestures. To be cut off from all physical contact is deeply painful. But Jesus broke into that man's universe of isolation with a single touch. So much love and grace went through that touch along with His healing power.

God blessings can continue to flow through us to touch the lives of people around us no matter what is going us in our lives.

When my husband and sons visited me, the nurses insisted that they must put on the green overall, face mask and wear the gloves. I strongly disagreed, stating that my family members lived in the same house with me where they were exposed to me and they touched me freely despite the affliction. There was no way I would agree to have my family especially my husband prohibited from touching me.

You cannot even begin to imagine how I waited in anticipation for my husband to visit and the joy that coursed through my heart when he stretched out his hand to touch me.

> *Room 217 at the end of the corridor*
> *May the magnificent views you give*
> *Of golden beams glowing over grey clouds*
> *Of the huge ball of fire descending*
> *behind snow-capped mountains*
> *Scattering fiery rays across the blue lake*
> *Cheer on your new occupants*
> *In the path to strength and health*

Ending 2011

Although 2011 was a very tough year because I had to deal with the isolation, reproach and loneliness that comes with long term chronic diseases, it was also a year many new things were birthed in my life. Without a voice and a physical audience, I began to express myself more in writing. It was amazing how the poetic muse began to ooze out from the depth of my pained heart. My Sista-friend BMM and my long-term mentee, Ojemsy encouraged me to explore the world of blogging. That was what I did. My sons pointed me in the direction of Google to find out how to set up a blog but my friend, Dewale assisted me to set it up. It took me a while to prepare my family and myself to share our lives in public. But I knew at the back of my heart that if the Lord wants to use my

> **Several times while I was in the hospital, the nurses talked about the fact that I was always smiling and singing despite the storms whirling around me.**

story to touch lives for good, then I had to be willing to be vulnerable. I had to be willing to let people see the painful path I was walking and how the Lord kept me through the path. I eventually posted my first blog on the November 1st, 2011. It was a Step of Faith as indicated in the title of the blog. My desire was that the story God is scripting of my life will touch lives for good and for His glory. That was the birth of my blog captioned "Enriching Lives, Inspiring Hope." The address was *TouchingLives4good*--that is what we prayed that each blog post would do; enrich lives, inspire hope and touch lives for good.

My gratitude knew no limit on Christmas day, counting my blessings and recounting the goodness of God in my life during the year despite all the challenges and difficult seasons we went through.

I determined that I don't have to see my breakthrough manifested before I am available to be used by God to bless others.

I had only three days to prepare after being away for over two weeks. I was grateful for the strength I had gained. We sang Christmas carols on Saturday night and enjoyed an uplifting fellowship with friends. Those timeless songs resonated the unchanging message of God's awesome love expressed in the giving of His precious Son to us.

With the same joyful spirit, we sang some more on Christmas day. We shared gifts of love, ate turkey and connected with families and friends all over the world. My Pastor in his sermon said, "God is a giving God"—this is the essence of Christmas. He gave His only begotten Son. He gave His best and most precious for us. He gave us the most precious Gift anyone could ever desire to have.

He did not hold back Him back--He gave Jesus up for us.Jesus gave up His glory and took the form of man. He gave His life to give us life. It reminded me of the chorus of the song – "I'm Forgiven" by the Imperials.

> *I'm forgiven*
> *Now I have a reason for living*
> *Jesus keeps giving and giving*
> *Giving till my heart overflows*

Jesus keeps giving and giving till my life overflows. He came to live and die so that we can live with Him in eternity. He gave to everyone who came to Him with a need. He gave without holding back. He gave freely, He gave completely and He gave His all. Truly the atmosphere was charged with the joy of sharing, giving and receiving love.

The cave of confinement squeezed gratitude out of me the way oil oozes from the crushed kernel pressed under pressure. It was in that cave, God shifted my focus from all that is around me to see His mighty hand at the top of the press and His other hand succouring me. Gratitude rolled away the heavy rock blocking the mouth of the cave. Gratitude led me out. But gratitude was a choice, a conscious determined choice.

#

Patiently Enduring With Joy

"Patience is not the ability to wait but how you act when you are waiting."

Patiently endure everything with joy--this was Paul's prayer in Colossians 1:11; "We ask him to strengthen you by his glorious might with all the power you need to patiently endure everything with joy." He knew we have need for strength from God to patiently endure challenging situations. As if that is not hard enough, He went further to pray that we would do it with joy.

Maintaining an attitude of joy in all circumstances, at all times and especially in hard and difficult situations, takes more than will power. It takes the grace of God. Throughout the course of the affliction that spanned over twenty years of my life, I found that the times that were most difficult for me to deal with were those times when I am alone in the hospital with no one to visit me and sometimes for days. It always seemed to be the last straw on top of an already heavy burden.

These were times when I was living in another country and my husband could not come to be with me or those times he had to go on official work-related trips while I was in the hospital. So far away from my home country and extended family, I felt very lonely often, and there were those times I actually felt abandoned. I missed my mother terribly at such times and the extended family structure we have back at home. There I know someone in the family or among friends will come and stay at my bedside especially when they know my husband is away.

It is especially during the long hospital stay when the ingredients to feel miserable are abundantly available and in the right proportion that I struggle a lot with enduring with joy at these times. The worst of these moments for me was during the hospital stay in Accra in May/June 2003. My husband had come to be with me and when it looked like things were getting better, he went back to Geneva to make necessary arrangements for us to come over when I got out of the hospital. He had barely gone when things took a turn for the worse. It was one of the worse moments of my life. I was struggling with the affliction and seemingly doing it alone, my husband could not get a reasonable flight back and I could not be with my children. They had to stay in the hotel and were not allowed into the high dependency ward I was in. I could only see them through the window.

Every day I saw the other patients surrounded by their families and friends during the visiting hours. The nurses kept asking me why I had no family to visit me. They forgot many times that I was not a Ghanaian and I was a staff of an International Organisation with few close friends in Accra at that time. I waited and waited during the visiting hours hoping and wishing someone would remember me and come for a visit. It is at those times that friends seem to have something important to do and could not just make it. I lost the battle with the struggle not to feel alone in the world and abandoned several times. Yet it was at one of such times as these that I was reminded to endure with joy and maintain a joyful attitude. I knew it had to start from within. I had to make a conscious effort and a choice either to sink into the pit of misery, anger, bitterness and loneliness or find something to be thankful to God for. It took conscious effort to swim against the direction of the tide. I knew that if I allowed myself to flow with the tide and with very strong undercurrent, the end result would be more anger, more bitterness and more pain. As I made the effort to focus my mind and my thoughts on reasons why I should be grateful for life, the tension always begins to ease. Singing songs of praise and just thanking God for who He is always lift me up and out of the pit. So I kept telling myself; "I've got joy of God in my heart" and kept singing:

> *I've got the joy of God in me x2*
> *I've got the spirit of the Son of God*
> *I've got the joy of God in me.*

Although I was not happy about the situation, slowly and surely joy rose from within my heart and gave me a reason to look beyond the misery around me to see God who is mindful of me in the place where I was at that moment. It is bad enough that I had to deal with the burden of the infirmity that has put me in the hospital and I may not be able to do anything about that situation. But I certainly could not allow the devil to steal my joy on top of this. That would be adding insult to the injury. I can do something about that, I can choose not to accept it.

No matter how difficult our lives' circumstances and challenges may be, the Word of God admonishes us to "count it all joy" because this trial of our faith will produce perseverance if we patiently endure to the end. Enduring means that it is something you rather not do but you are encouraged to do it. The pressured times in our lives are like the processing that every raw material must go through so that a great and high quality product can be made of out them. Focusing my attention on these truths often helps to give me the much needed impetus to be thankful, full of praise and move towards being joyful even when it seems most difficult.

#

Keep Hope Alive

Finding a reason to get out of bed each day became hard and difficult. The only motivation sometimes was the fact that I knew someone is waiting along this hard road to light his candle from mine. I know someone is waiting at the end of the dark tunnel to receive an encouragement or comfort that I have received if I could just push right through to the end. Because all of the experiences I have gone through is not about me alone. All of these certainly could not be just about me. There is a reason why God told me He would comfort me in all my trials with the same comfort with which I would comfort others in their trials and afflictions. All of these must be about the lives God wants to use my story to touch.

One day I was full of life and strength. The next day the symptoms returned with the fury of a wounded animal as if to challenge my right to live and enjoy life to the full. At such times, it is easy to throw up my arms over my head and bow in despair. It is easy to wail and bemoan the situation like one without a glimmer of hope. Or how do you live each day in the fear of what may and can happen next?

The swiftness with which the situation changed often left me giddy. Just when I least expected, another discovery was made - a diagnosis that threw me off balance. In a twinkling of an eye, all I have planned for that period spiraled out of control as doctors call for more tests and investigation. As if it was not bad enough to deal with the respiratory and neuromuscular diseases, the doctors found out that I was having pulmonary hypertension. The respiratory disease with the attending complications was putting pressure on my heart forcing it to pump more than normal. New drugs had to be added to the long list of drugs I was taking. My doctors insisted that I must rest my heart by using the ventilator more frequently not just in the night, but also during the day.

Tears laced my lower eyes lids when my husband got the bill for the new drugs. It would cost us an additional 6000.00 Swiss Francs per month to purchase this drug, which the doctors insisted I must use regularly to control the pulmonary hypertension. "Is there no end to this?" my heart cried out in anguish, "this is just too much for one person to bear."

I could not afford to give up on hope. To lose hope is to fall into the pit of despair and depression. Hopelessness makes men desperate, desperate people do desperate things and it never ends well. It is not a good place to be when a man cannot find a reason not to give in or a reason not to give up. When a man loses hope, he loses all reasons to live. I have a reason to live. I have my husband. I have my two sons. I have dreams waiting to be accomplished and lived. Hopelessness brings heaviness to the spirit and causes depression but God strengthens the heart of those who hope in Him. I purposed in heart to be strong and take heart because I put hope in the God. I could not have survived the ordeal without the hope that only Jesus gives. My hope hinged on nothing else but Jesus Christ.

I was not without hope. In the ferocious whirlwind of affliction, hope kept me anchored on the solid rock of ages. I had to find purpose in the whirlwind that could keep me grounded, and not swirled or tossed around. God's mercy had kept me thus so far, so

I could not afford to let go at this point. I chose to cling tenaciously to my hope in God which is able to keep me going through the tough seasons.

One day, I was in the bathroom following a severe bout of coughing. I had brought up so much awful secretion that I needed to rinse my mouth and also empty my bladder. As I washed my hands in the basin I looked up and saw a scary image in the mirror staring back at me. The skin was drawn across my cheekbones. The strain of breathing was conspicuously visible. The person in the mirror was looking so gaunt I could not recognize her but for the purple Chinese - styled pyjamas top she was wearing. I took a long look at the stranger in the mirror and I began to speak the Word of God, the word of life to her. I spoke to her as I would speak to someone standing in front of me. I told her she is restored. I told her she would live to declare the glory of God.

From that day on, I began to say to myself all the things I would have said to someone else going through a tough time and in adversity. I needed to hear my own sermon. I told myself what hope means. It means to look beyond the cloud of despair and see a silver lining. It means I would choose not to complain about what was going on but I will trust in God's providence to change the situation for the better, if it pleases Him. Though, I didn't how He was going to do it and I didn't understand why I have to deal with all of these issues.

How was it possible to stay calm and steadfast in the season of pain and distress? How can it be possible to be at peace in the inner mind and at rest in the midst of this storm? Can one possibly get to the point where one's life will model the quiet confidence of one who knows that his/her heavenly Father knows what He is doing, and that He has your back? I knew He would surely not stand aside and watch me suffer without a reason. David encouraged himself in the Lord in the time of great distress and adversity when the Amalekites ravaged their town and took away all their wives, children and properties. I borrowed a leaf from David and began to encourage myself in the Lord. I told myself that since I am still alive by the grace and mercy of God, then there is hope for me. While there is life, there is hope that things will turn around for my good. I rested on the assurance that hope brought me. So I will rest on the Solid Rock of impregnable strength, who would never fail me or let me fall to the ground or the swept away by the force of the furious whirlwind. Learning to be quiet and at peace amid of the turbulence became a daily lesson.

God who knows it all knows it best. The All-knowing God knows what is best in every situation and circumstances. The assurance of this knowledge and my experience of God became a strong anchor for my hope

At such times when we are visited by the storms of life, God calls out to us to fall back on Him. He promises to catch us and save us from falling. Yet one of the most difficult thing to do is to rest, lean on and totally depend on God to take care of us. When we are unsure and things are uncertain, learning to trust and obey God becomes an imperative.

\#

In The Waiting Room

The waiting room—the place where you learn to hold on to the Word of God as if you next breath depends on it--the place where the Word becomes to you a life line.

Waiting in any form can be tough but it is essential.

What are you waiting for – a change, a breakthrough, an answer to a prayer or a miracle?

Whatever it is, you can rejoice in the waiting room because God knows you are there.

God takes note. He hears your deep, silent and unspoken cry. He notices you.

I simply love God. He works in amazing ways to assure you that He knows you are in the waiting room. Sometimes He sends His servants to confirm His Word just for you to know that He takes note of all that concerns you. He is God of knowledge. He knows where you are.

I had testified of how God restored my strength and enabled me to do a number of things I had not been able to do for a long while. Barely a week afterward, I noticed the symptoms returned with fury. At first, I ignored it; I told myself I don't have to accept its presence or message. I chose to focus on the truth, and that is – I am healed and I am delivered from the harassment of the affliction.

Within a few more days, my condition got worse, I was struggling and I was angry but I knew I had to turn my energy again to wage warfare against this encroachment on my health. One night, distressed with the choking, head resting on my hands, elbows burrowed into my laps, I sat on my bed and declared, "Thank You God, thank You because I have hope, thank You that I know Your promises concerning me." I knew that without this assurance holding my heart trusting in the Lord, the cloud of heaviness and despair would envelop me. I asked God for a peaceful night's rest, standing on the authority of His word – He gives His beloved sleep. I am His beloved. I am precious in His sight. I slept through the night.

The following morning God confirmed that He has His eyes on me in the waiting room. He sent me a message through His servant – a phone call from a dear Sister who declared to me the Word God placed on her heart concerning me. It was timely and on target. I was overwhelmed. It got to me the way God assured me that He takes notice of me. He is taking note of every detail of my life – what I was doing in His service, what I was struggling with and what I was going through. Nothing about me was hidden from Him. In a flash, the cloud of despair dissipated and my spirit was elated.

Be assured, dear friend, God takes notice of you in the waiting room. He will confirm His Word to you in mysterious ways. So while you are waiting you can draw on the infinite reservoir of His grace. You can make your time in the waiting room worthwhile by being busy doing good. You can let the time count for something of eternal value.

Your waiting time is a time to nourish the seed you have planted – with praise, with prayer, and with abundant patience.

Your waiting room can become the presence room where you wait in the presence of God to comfort and strengthen you, the place where you can experientially declare, "Thou art with me." It can be a time of refreshing and renewal in His presence.

While Joseph was waiting for his dream to come true, he maintained an exemplary character in the face of temptation, he was an excellent worker in the prison and he was attentive to the needs of others. He used the gifts and talents God blessed him with to meet the need of others. And he was still waiting for his heart desire to be fulfilled. You too have been blessed with a gift, a talent or a skill which can be used to bless lives around you while you are waiting. There is something in your hands you can release to be used of God to add value to the lives of others. Everyone has something in their hands – no one is empty handed. Give and be assured that God will honour His word.

> To you, my dear friend in the waiting room, I write:
> Be at rest. Let His peace enfold you.
> Be creative, be passionate and be zealous at doing good.
> Wait with hope. Wait with expectation.
> Wait with patience. Wait trusting in God. Wait doing good.

Though things may be contrary to your dream and desire now, don't give up, don't give in, hold on tenaciously to your dream and give it all you have got.

Watch out for God. Be attentive to hear His voice and the confirmation of His everlasting love for you.

When and how will it end?

I can't give an answer, but this much I know, it will be a demonstration of the sovereignty of God and a display of His power at work in you. For Joseph, it happened – at that moment, in a flash – the years of waiting were wiped out.

For you too, the end point will bear God's signature if you wait on God.

#

Investment of Eternal Value

"No one is more cherished in this world than someone who lightens the burden of another" - Author Unknown.

In previous sections, I wrote about how we can keep hope alive especially when we are "In the Waiting Room." In this chapter, I want to expand more on investing in the lives of others. This is applicable to everyone and not only those in the waiting room. Investing in lives is making deposits of our resources — time, energy and sometimes finances — into the lives of others. Not as to receive a high return here but to add value of eternal significance to their lives. I quite honestly believe that doing this when the natural response to our circumstances is to be dejected and morose makes the devil mad.

One verse in the Bible motivates me to strive to be a conduit of God's blessings come what may and irrespective of my circumstances. It is, "I will make you into a great nation. I will bless you and make you famous, and you will be a blessing to others." (Gen 12:2). In blessing Abram, God desired for him to be a dispenser of good and a conduit of His blessings to others. That is one of my deepest heart desires; to be an inexhaustible dispenser of good no matter what estate of life I may be in.

As God truly blessed Abraham so that he could be a blessing to others so also has He blessed each of us His children to be a blessing. God blessings can continue to flow through us to touch the lives of people around us no matter what is going us in our lives. Those things going on should not turn us into dams or reservoirs of God's blessings.

We are not conduits of God's blessings only when things are going great for us and when we have more than enough. We are called to be continually conduits of God's blessings irrespective of the challenges we face in life or the adversity we go through. These difficult situations should not make us any less generous. The widow who willingly made a cake of bread for Elijah with the little flour and oil she had left, did so in an austere and difficult times. And there was food for her, her son and Elijah every day afterward.

There is nothing more that matters to me after my salvation and my family than to ensure that my life touches lives for good and that I am able to impact lives of those around me in such a way that it would leave an echo that will continue to resound long after I have gone. I also think we can make the devil mad by going around doing good, even when he is going out of his way to harass us and making every attempt to ensure that we lose our joy and peace. Some of the ways that we can do good to others and invest in the lives of others do not need more than a conscious decision to do so on our part.

Several times while I was in the hospital, the nurses talked about the fact that I was always smiling and singing despite the storms whirling around me. It gladdened my heart to know that the smile and the singing made a little difference in lifting up the spirit of those around me. Smiling when your circumstances dictate otherwise radiates your confidence in God and His glory to those around you.

I also learnt that seeking opportunities to do something that will impact someone's life for good—deliberately sowing seeds of goodness into the life of someone brought into my life helped me to focus on others and take my attention off what I was going through.

"Everyone deserves someone who will make them look forward to tomorrow" – this is a quote by an unknown author. This is what an encourager does, he/she gives others reasons not to give up but to hold on to God Who makes all things beautiful in His own time. You can be the person whose words will lighten up someone's face and give them a reason to go on. This is one that I know God gave me the grace to do. I soon realize that despite the difficult challenges I was going through, I could still give words of encouragement to others.

Seeking opportunities to be a conduit of God's blessing to others helped me to take my eyes off the storm raging around me. It is my earnest desire to be the bearer of God's answer to someone's prayer. Joseph has remained a very good example for me in this regard. He did not hesitate to interpret the dreams of others when he was still waiting for his own dream to come through. He was willing to invest in others and be a blessing to them while he was waiting for his heart desire to be manifested. I determined that I don't have to see my breakthrough manifested before I am available to be used by God to bless others.

#

In Desperate Need of Relief

While I have talked about the many battles I faced in the hospitals and in my mind, it would be remiss of me to exclude this particular incident which would have seen me addicted or seeking solace outside of Jesus.

I awoke to the claws of the cough clutching my chest. Pain and anguish ensnared my body. In distress, I cried out to the Lord. I found no rest or comfort sitting, lying down or standing. Often bent over, I groaned, "Lord, deliver me from this cough." My breath was short as the cough cut off my breath. My throat was hoarse and patched like one lost in a hot dry desert where there is no water. Water offered no respite nor did it soothe my throat. It merely filled my bladder and sent me off to the bathroom.

I was at this point ready to do anything for a break, for a relief and for a respite. That was when I began to think about alcohol. I thought perhaps if I could have a cup of tea laced with brandy or rum, it would soothe my throat from the throbbing intensity of the long-drawn out coughing episodes. I began to imagine the warmth of the alcohol heated up in hot tea seeping into the soreness of my throat and radiating into my hurting chest. But I had no brandy or rum. I am not even a social drinker. I have abstained from drinking for almost three decades. I have very low tolerance for alcohol. A cup of wine was enough to get me singing like a canary, reducing my inhibition. I also had the personal conviction that the Bible asked us to exercise caution with alcohol.

I told my husband I wished I was still actively baking and I had a bottle of brandy at home. I used the brandy to preserve and flavour my cake especially when I use fruits in the cake. I tried to convince him that the tea laced with alcohol would bring me the much-needed relief. I thought I could get him to go and get the small sachets from the *Tabac*, the corner shops in the city. He reminded me we don't drink alcohol and he did not think alcohol was what I needed.

The desperate longing for alcohol shocked me. I could not believe how much I wanted the relief I felt the drink would bring me. Since I was without the option of the alcohol laced tea, and the hot tea my husband offered at that point in time did not fit into kind of relief I imagined alcohol would offer me, I knew I had to be relentless in my crying to God for relief. I just wanted God to knock me out so that I would not feel any more pain or distress. I wanted Him to put me out of the misery that so strongly overwhelmed me. It was during those times that I wept before the Lord, "Father, wrap Your mighty hands around me, and let the warmth of Your breath soothe my pain."

My cry went up into the heavens into His ears. He heard my cry and harkened to my voice. His peace enveloped me. As a mother singing a lullaby to her fretting child, I imagined the sound of His heartbeat lulling me into a deep sleep. The next thing I saw was the light of a new day streaming through the partially closed shutters. The dark night had passed. It was the dawn of a new day.

A couple of years after this incident, I read Proverbs 31:6 during a study of the Book of Proverbs. I read the verse in Amplified and The Message Version.

"Give strong drink (as medicine) to him who is ready to pass away, and wine to him in bitter distress of heart." (AMP)

"Use wine and beer only as sedatives, to kill the pain and dull the ache of the terminally ill, for whom life is a living death." (MSG)

Let him drink and remember his misery no more.

That was when I remembered my desperate longing for alcohol-laced tea. I understood the depth of misery that would necessitate the recommendation from the Bible to give alcohol to relieve pain or distress. I understood how one could desperately desire alcohol at such a low point when pain becomes so overwhelming and unbearable.

It is so sweet to have Jesus to trust in and to be able to take Him at His word. It is wonderful to have His promises to hold on to. It was at such times that I wondered how people who do not have hope or trust in the Lord go through adversity. I can now understand why many would slip into depression or become alcoholics. Without doubt, if we had had alcohol at home and if my husband had not exercised restraint by refusing to consider that option, I would have gone down that slippery slope to find help where there is no lasting help. Without that option on the plate, I was compelled to stay focused on God the ultimate Helper of the helpless, and He did not disappoint me. He came through for me again and again.

My Journey in Pictures

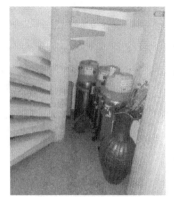
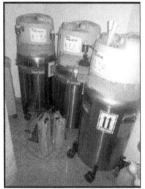

Oxygen reservoir

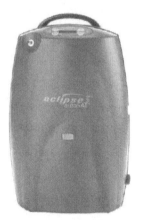
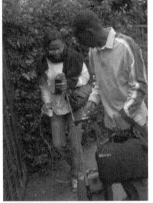

Husband helping with oxygen
concentrator-2009

Eclipse oxygen concentrator for travels

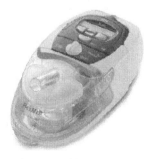
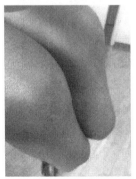

resmed-cpap-machines

Legs after amputation

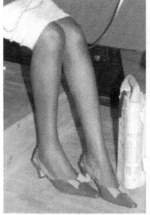

Legs before amputation

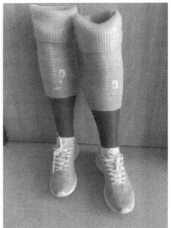

The New Prostethic Leg

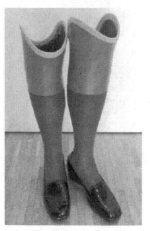

The New Prostethic Leg

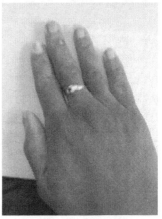

Hand with necrosis and damaged nails

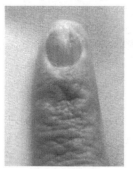

Nail deformed

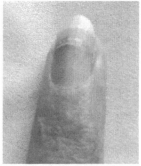

My Nails Post Operation

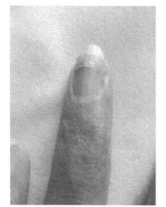
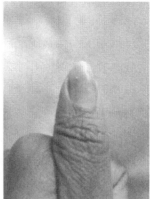

My Nails Post Operation

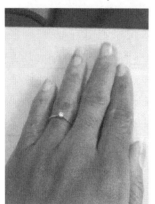
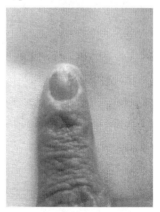

Hands with necrosis and damaged nails

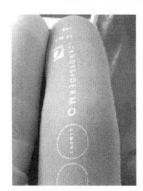
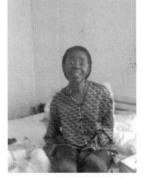

Post Operation Delighted to
Be Alive

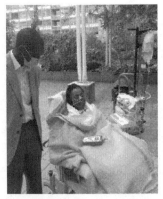
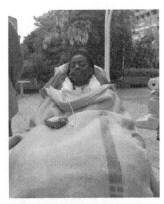

The day before amputation on the terrace

One day before Surgery 2

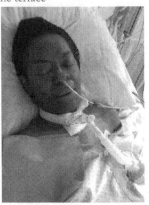

On the hospital Bed and Hooked up to the Oxygen Machine

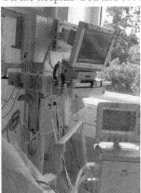
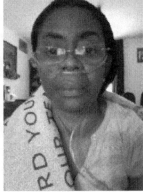

Machines I was connected to

With healing verses blanket. Speaking My Faith

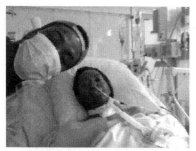

ICU-HUG post transplant with Ose

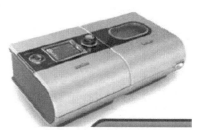

resmed cpap_medium

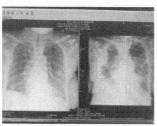

Lungs Before Transplant

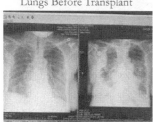

Lungs days and 4 weeks after transplantation

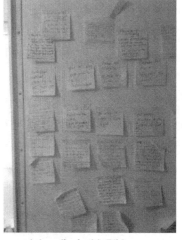

post-it inscribed with Bible verses on my wardrobe door

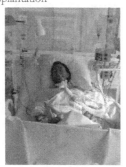

ICU-HUG post transplant

PART THREE

The Epic
STORM

The Storm Hits

2013

The gale force wind that unleashed its fury on us in January 2013 began brewing in September 2012 when I noticed a pronounced swelling at the right side of my neck just above my clavicle. At first, I thought it was because of the forceful and incessant coughing. I had noticed the ballooning around the base of my neck when coughing. I noticed the enlarging of vein. Towards the end of September, we realized this was no ordinary swelling resulting from the cough. My doctors began to investigate the swelling. I underwent several tests and procedure to determine what the swell was. On one occasion, they attempted to aspirate the swelling. The procedure failed at the first attempt. I did a scintillography and a biopsy of the cyst to ascertain whether the cyst was malignant. I could not thank God enough when the results came back and it was a benign cyst.

The cyst was growing rapidly causing concerns that it could grow inward and block my air passage. The doctors began to discuss the possibilities for removing it. We learnt fast that it would be difficult to remove the cyst under general anaesthesia. The state of my lungs made intubation risky as the anaesthetist may not be able to bring me out of sleep after the surgery. The only option was to remove it under local anaesthesia, which the doctors deemed would be very painful and distressing.

By the second week of December, the cyst had become so big that I needed a scarf to cover my neck. It was like a one-sided goitre. Another attempt was made to aspirate the fluid in the cyst. It was successful. They drained a large quantity of the fluid and the size was reduced significantly. Within one week of this procedure, the cyst began to grow again, this time at a faster rate. By Christmas, it was back to its former size. I had to call the hospital on the 27th of December and went back to see my doctor. There was no point trying to aspirate the fluids. The decision was taken to remove it immediately after the holidays in January 2016.

I crossed over into the New Year, looking up to God and asking Him to bring a turnaround for good for me. The strain of the cough and the difficulties in breathing was sapping my strength. Little did I know that there was an epic storm on the way. The dark black clouds of this storm will for a period obscure the sunlight of my life. And the force of the gale winds would be strong enough to break branches off my body. Nothing prepared me for the aftermath of this epic storm. It simply left me stunned.

#

A Stormy Beginning

I arrived in the hospital on the morning of January 2nd, 2013 for the procedure to remove the fast-growing cyst on my neck. We had anticipated that the procedure would be performed that morning but that was not the case. The surgeon had to attend to several emergencies. They came later in the evening to explain to me how they would perform the surgery under local anaesthetics. They wanted me to know that they will do everything possible to minimize the distress. But the location of the cyst would require that my neck be extended backward to facilitate the procedure, which would not be a comfortable position.

When I was wheeled into the theatre the following morning, I was actively praying and asking God for the grace to go through the procedure. It was indeed a test of endurance--how much pain, distress and discomfort I could gracefully endure. Note that I said gracefully endure. I wondered how I would go through what they had told me would be a very painful procedure without screaming out. They had to fix the ventilator to facilitate my breathing in a way that would not disturb the work of the surgeons. Someone had to manually hold the cap over my face throughout the procedure. The pressure of this doctor's hands over my face added to the distress. I asked the Lord to hold my right hand and surround me with His presence. He did. He held my hands throughout the surgery and kept me from being overtaken by distress.

> I asked the Lord to hold my right hand and surround me with His presence. He did. He held my hands throughout the surgery and kept me from being overtaken by distress.

Transferring me from the theatre to the recovery room was an ordeal. They had to use another ventilator that was battery powered. The pressure delivered by the ventilator was different; I could not breathe properly with it. The short distance between the theatre and the recovery room felt like a mile long. I was gasping for breath by the time I got to the recovery room and frantically gesticulating to the attendants to change the ventilators as fast as they could to the one I was familiar with. I overhead the attending nursing saying that I could hardly wait to have my ventilator back on.

Hours later, the doctors said, "Madame Olumese, you were brave and courageous." I mustered the strength to smile and give thanks to God Who held me in His Hands. I spent the night in the Intensive Care Unit. By this time, I had lost count of the number of times I had been in this ICU. It had become a familiar environment.

> "I can't take any more." That was what was going on inside me. Yet what came out was a soft whisper, "Give me the grace to endure this night, Lord."

That night was one of the longest in my life. The pain swept over me in waves. I could not find a single position that was comfortable. I wanted to scream, "I can't take any more." That was what was going on inside me. Yet what came out was a soft whisper, "Give me the grace to endure this night, Lord."

And the night did pass because the covenant-keeping faithfulness of God endures forever. With the dawn of the new day came the assurance of hope and confirmation of the victory God wrought for me. I welcomed the light of the new day filtering through a side window. This year had to hold more for me inspite of this stormy beginning. I was desperate for a turn around. I needed a change in this status quo.

I fixed my gaze on God, who only is able to deliver me. The wait continued. And the storm gathered strength on the horizon.

#

Standing Against The Old Prophet

Two years and two months after my first encounter with the Old Prophet I met him again in January 2013. I had been recalled to the hospital in Lausanne to see if there had been any changes in my status. The team in Geneva had hinted that I had moved up on the waiting list and it was appropriate to have this check-up. I found that I had to stay in the hospital for three days and all the tests I had done before were repeated. It was at the end of the battery of tests and investigations that the *Old Prophet* came to see me. It was in the evening. I was in bed. He came into the room in his white coat and stood over my bed. He was relentless in his quest to paint a picture of a hopeless situation. He thought it was my right to be fully informed. He again described the complexity of the situation and called them a constellation of risks. He was so explicit and graphic in presenting the picture that if it were not for the peace of God guarding my heart, it would have melted in fear. In the audacity of arrogance, he displayed, he wanted my approval for his position.

> **No *Old Prophet* will deprive me the opportunity to live the life that God has given me. Too much had been taken from me, I would not allow this opportunity to taken from me without a fight.**

He saw no hope. He offered no hope. He stripped all hope away.

I wondered what he wanted from me; to jump off the cliff and put an end to it right away or resign myself to fate and wait for death to catch up on me?

A Yoruba adage says, one death cannot kill the same person twice! I was not going to let it happen again. Suddenly, something welled up in my heart against him and there was a strong nudging in my spirit to resist him. I knew I had to take charge of the situation. The tone of my voice changed. I felt like I grew taller in my spirit and he was no longer looming over me. I refused to be cowered by his words. I knew at that instant that we were not wrestling against flesh and blood in this matter but against spiritual wickedness in high places. I refused to be pushed over the edge into the pit of despair and fear. God gave me the grace and the strength to challenge him. I looked him straight in the eye and told him that if medical science had no other option to offer me that I was going to take what was available to me despite the risks involved. Even if it was time for me to go home, it would not be out of fear and not because I did not do all that was required of me but because God says it is time. No *Old Prophet* will deprive me the opportunity to live the life that God has given me. Too much had been taken from me, I would not allow this opportunity to taken from me without a fight.

I felt that if we cannot offer a glimmer of hope, we should not extinguish whatever hope the person had left. Our words should not leave people in despair and without a hope.

"Raise a clarion call" rang loud and clear in my spirit and I knew what we had to do.

My husband walked into the room as the Old Prophet prepared to leave. He had no further response to my position. After he left us, I shared all that transpired with my husband who began to thank God for the peace with which He garrisoned our hearts against agitating fears. Our hearts were at peace trusting in the Lord and we were not moved. It was pure joy to stumble on Psalm 108: 1-6 later that night as I flipped through the Bible in search of something to read.

"O God, my heart is fixed - steadfast in the confidence of faith. Therefore, I will praise and make melody. I am God's beloved. He will answer me and deliver me." (Psalm 57:7, 108:1,6 - *paraphrased*). I was glad that I knew experientially and beforehand that I would see the goodness of God in the land of the living. It gave me such a reassuring confidence to have this awesome promise.

At The Precipice of Despair

The following day, I met some other members of the *Old Prophet's* team. When they came in, they sat down. They did not stand over me. They presented the same information, even as graphic as the Old Prophet did. But with each challenge, they offered a possible solution. They offered no guarantee, but they gave hope. They were committed to finding a way around each obstacle facing us to the best of their ability.

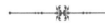

When your faith is established in the Lord and your heart is stayed on God, only then will you be able to sing and praise God in anticipation of what God will do irrespective of the situation.

It was the "same information, different presentation, different attitude, different result. When they left, they did not leave me in despair. They left me with some degree of assurance. It was at that point that I began to ponder on how our words can affect the lives of people we encounter. I wondered if we take care to ensure that our words are full of life, hope and encouragement. I wondered if we understood that when we are not mindful of our words, we can use our words to sow seeds of discouragement and strip away hope from our listeners with our words just as the Old prophet would have used his words to strip away hope from me if not for the grace and mercies of God.

You also can find a promise in the word of God to fix your gaze upon and to keep you from slipping into the pit of despair and hopelessness.

I felt that if we cannot offer a glimmer of hope, we should not extinguish whatever hope the person had left. Our words should not leave people in despair and without a hope. I re-committed myself from that day to be an encourager at every instance as the Lord gives me the grace. I will be careful never to allow my words strip anyone of hope. Even when I have to present hard truths or facts, I will do my best to find a way to present them with an assurance of a way out. There will be times when we will be duty-bound to present a grim picture but we must not do so in a way that will put the receiver of that information at the precipice of despair.

This can be as subtle as the comments we make on issues concerning our nations, our families, our workplace (bosses), our churches, etc. The degree of hopelessness that is sometimes transmitted by comments people carelessly make can be heart-breaking. I believe that we must be mindful not to extinguish hope with our words but to ignite hope.

Perhaps at this time you are also in a deep and complex situation where the problems are multi-dimensional and there seems to be no solution in sight. You are overwhelmed by many afflictions and pressed down by loads of care. Your heart is aching. You pine and long for a resolution and a change in the situation. It is possible that you may be at the brink of despair at this time. At such times, at the precipice of despair, we need a Friend. We must be very sure our anchor holds on a solid rock and our hearts are fixed on confident assurance that we have a Saviour Who can move the mountain. I encourage you to pause from reading and ponder on God's promise for you as relates to what you may be going through. I beseech you to let His promise seep into your spirit and take root there. I encourage you to hold on, cling to hope, don't give up. God will surely come through for you. Let your heart be fixed trusting in His unfailing love for you.

Mountains may shake, earth may quake, and the storms may swirl furiously, cling to hope. Let your heart be steadfast and confident. When your faith is established in the Lord and your heart is stayed on God, only then will you be able to sing and praise God in anticipation of what God will do irrespective of the situation. This brings hope. But if only in this world we have a hope, we will be of all men most miserable. If by the abounding grace of God, we are able to maintain a composed frame of mind in the midst of the crisis, we have an even greater reason to be full of praise and to be thankful. Though the change we long for may seem long in coming but if we pay attention, we will see His mighty hand holding us up. For this again, we can be thankful.

> I chose to live and I chose to fight for life; knowing fully well that my weapon of warfare is not carnal but mighty through God, to knock down the strongholds of human reasoning and to destroy false arguments.

There is the card I wrote and pasted on my wardrobe door in 2008. I placed it in the line of my vision when I used to sit at the edge of the bed on my hands. It was Psalm 108:1. I placed it there to remind myself that my heart must remain fixed, steadfast and confident in the Lord despite the billows roaring around me.

"My heart, O God, is steadfast (fixed); I will sing and make music with all my soul." (**Paraphrased**)

You also can find a promise in the word of God to fix your gaze upon and to keep you from slipping into the pit of despair and hopelessness.

#

Caught In The Middle

At the end of the three-day sojourn in the hospital in Lausanne, I returned home knowing that the battle line had been drawn and I could not afford to be lethargic or lackadaisical about this battle. The battle was not one I could fight in the physical. It was one to be fought on my knees. I knew I could not afford offense to take root in my heart. If I allow myself to focus on the attitude of the Old Prophet, I would lose the battle upfront. That was a risk I was not prepared to take. There was a switch in my mind set--I had to be battle ready. I took my position at the front line and was ready to fight for a chance to live.

The following day, I called Dr. PG to inform her of what transpired at the Hospital in Lausanne. To say that she was livid would put it mildly. I was expected to have gone for a check-up visit not for a full blown work-up. It was apparent that this was contrary to usual practice. By the time I relayed the entire incidence, I knew she was going to take it up at the meeting with the Transplant Team.

It was at my next appointment with the Geneva Team lead by Dr. PG that I got the indication of the intensity of discussions held over my case. As a Senior colleague, the Old Prophet positioned himself against me and proposed that I should be removed from the waiting list for transplantation. He was convinced that I was not a suitable candidate. The Geneva team were angry that the full work-up was undertaken without their being informed and without their consent. It was perceived as the Old Prophet using his seniority to undermine the Geneva team who are my immediate physicians and most cognisant of my state of health.

I learnt as I pieced together the several bits of information slipping through that the two camps were pitched against each other and I was caught in the middle of the crossfire. So I decided to take the battle to the level where I knew I have been equipped to wield power and authority. I refused to be a victim of the battle. I refused to be a collateral damage. Creflo Dollar once told a woman stricken with cancer, "woman, choose to live!" I chose to live and I chose to fight for life; knowing fully well that my weapon of warfare is not carnal but mighty through God, to knock down the strongholds of human reasoning and to destroy false arguments. I could not align my thoughts with the false arguments that was promoting death for me. I had to align my thoughts with the truth of the word of God that promised me abundant life.

The Call

It was a phone call...
Long awaited phone call...

It came when least expected on Saturday, April 13th, 2013.

I was deep in the middle of the preparation for a Women's Seminar in church, an event I was looking forward to with great expectation. My SistaFriend, Bidemi, was coming to Geneva. It would be our first time of meeting in the flesh. Her book, Sistapower, was to be launched during the Women's Seminar. At the onset of the preparations, my husband advised me to actively involve other women in church in the organising of the event. I did. The two female pastors in church were in my house the previous Saturday and we went over every single detail of the event scheduled for April 27th. During the week following the meeting I found myself making a list of everything that was needed to be done and where what would be needed were kept. I even brought out the balloons to be used and the pump I hired for use. I indicated in my list where the balloon pump was to go after the event. I am a detailed planner but never this organised that early in advance of an event. I was driven by an inexplicable sense of urgency.

It was exactly two weeks to the event. My husband had just left for the usual Saturday Choir practice in church. I sat down on the black sofa by the bookshelf going over my list of things to do. I wanted to cross-check several things before going to rest on the ventilator as advised by my husband before he left. My son, Ehi was home with me. I was not doing very well, hence the need for the rest.

The phone rang. It must have been around 4:00pm.

The handset was not by my side. I got up to pick it from the centre table.

"Hello..."
"Madame Olumese?"
"Yes, this is Irene."
"My name is Prof. R.'
I knew who he was. I knew also that it was not a social call.

"We are ready for you..."

I did not hear much of what he said, my mind had wandered far away. I knew what had happened. There was someone waiting on a life support machine to give me a priceless gift, someone I will never know or be able to thank was gone. A family was in sorrow because someone had paid the ultimate price for me to have this precious gift. A wave of panic swept through me.

"Are you ready?" He asked. I guessed he wondered when he did not get a response from me.

My heart skipped a beat and began to race. Panic...

I slowly lowered myself back on the sofa. My legs were about to give way under me. I could feel every pounding of my heart on my temple.

"Am I ready? Irene, what have you let yourself into?" That was the thought that flashed in my mind. And my heart turned to a blob of melted wax within me.

It took every ounce of strength I could muster to mutter a weak "Yes"

He asked me if there had been any change of note in my health status since my last appointment. I responded in the negative.

"See you in the hospital," with that he signed off. It was the Head of Pulmonology unit in the Teaching Hospital who had called. He was the one on call that weekend in the Transplant Unit charged with the responsibility of informing patients on the waiting list when a donor becomes available.

Panic. Panic... Panic...I sat there on the sofa and tried to calm myself down.

"God, now? Two weeks to SistaPower Seminar? You are in control," I whispered in prayer. I was shaking all over. Wave after wave of panic swept over me. I felt light headed and it happened again. I knew it was coming and I could not hold it back. My bladder opened up. Thankfully, I had emptied my bladder a short-while earlier, so my bladder was not full. I lifted myself out of the chair and went into the guest bathroom. I called my son to come down from his room. I asked him to bring me another pair of trousers and the ventilator. I was struggling to breathe. The panic attack was making breathing difficult. It was from the bathroom I called my husband, his phone rang but he did not pick up. No surprise there. I knew he must have put it on silence when he started the choir practice. I asked my son to start calling one member of the choir after the other with the hope that someone had his phone on. We got the pianist. I asked him to give the phone to my husband.

"Honey, they called from the hospital. Prof. R. just called." He knew what that meant. We had waited over two years for that call but when it came I was least prepared for it.

"I am on my way home." He dropped the phone. Then I got a call from the Transplant Central Unit to notify me that they were sending an ambulance for me. I told them my husband would bring me in. I didn't want the ambulance to come before my husband arrived or before we had time to process what was about to happen. I called my husband back, this time he was in the car on his way home. I told him about the ambulance and he asked me to call them back that they should come. The centre for the transplant is 60km from Geneva and he knew there would be traffic on a Saturday evening.

While waiting for my husband to arrive back at home. I got on the ventilator. I needed to stop my heart rate from rising. I asked Ehi to call his brother, Ose, in the university in the United States. He got him right away. He was not at a basketball game or practice or anywhere where he could not answer the phone. Ehi said Ose answered the phone, he told him that I had been called to the hospital for the transplant. Ose answered, "uh hm!" and dropped the phone. It was much later that I learnt that he was sleeping when his brother called him. He recalled answering and going straight back to sleep. Then he jumped out of sleep with a start when the news registered. He called back immediately. I spoke with him. I asked him to go and stay with his Pastor or Bible study leader. I did not want him to be alone while waiting for the surgery to be over. It was going to be a long night on our side and a long day for him.

We called our close family friend, Mayor, he was on the list of those upholding us in prayer. We needed him to come and drive Ehi after us to the hospital. He got on his way in that instant. Then we had the ambulance pulled into our driveway and the panic began all over again.

"Constellation of risks" echoed from a distance in my mind. "Lord, please help me," I prayed silently. The ventilator mask was over my face and my heart sped up.

My husband went down to meet the ambulance-men and brought them up. They measured my vital signs and prepared me to go. They wanted to know if I could walk downstairs or they needed to carry me as the stretcher could not come up my spiral stairway. I told them I could and took off the ventilator mask. It was a slow walk down the stairway. My mind was blank. I was helped to get on the stretcher and was wheeled into the ambulance. They strapped me down and placed me back on the ventilator while my husband got in front beside the driver. Once we were settled, the driver backed out of our driveway, the siren came on and the vehicle turned left into Les Fayards Road and sped towards Lausanne. The speed was unnerving. I wanted the driver to take his time. I was not in a hurry to get there. I kept thinking about my unknown benefactor and wondering what the family must be going through at that time.

The kilometres between my house and the hospital disappeared fast. We were soon in Lausanne. The driver slowed down slightly as he drove through the city to the hospital. We got to the hospital and I was taken into the emergency room. The nurses came to go over the preparatory procedures with me. I had to change into the theatre gown. I got off the bed and stood up as my husband helped me to undress and removed my trousers. The nurses were ready to take me in and my son was still on the way. I wanted to see him before I was taken in but they would not wait.

I remember praying and asking God to hold me in His Hands. I remember telling my husband that whatever happened the SistaPower Seminar must go on.

"I will be back." I promised my husband as I was wheeled away from him down the corridor to the theatre. He was not allowed to follow. I could not look back to see his face.

#

The Valley of the Shadow of Death

My next recollection was on a day I thought was April 22nd when I told the nurse that the following day was my 21st wedding anniversary. From the bits and pieces of information I could put together of the events that transpired during that period, that scene was impossible; it took place in my subconscious.

I was told that the surgery itself went very well. The surgeons finished the transplantation in the early hours of April 14th. None of the "constellation of risks" that was envisaged happened during the surgery. Less than 48 hours after the surgery though, I was told that I developed complications that were severe enough for medical coma to be induced. I was in that state for four weeks. I learnt I was on a heart-lung machine (extracorporeal membrane oxygenation), haemodialysis and ventilator, to sustain my systems during this period.

My husband is the best person to recount all the events that took place during the time I was in coma. My experience of that time was different. I will share that in the next chapter. It took me a while to work out the timeline of all that took place during that period. He was very scanty with the information. I asked everyone who had the opportunity to visit to tell me what they saw. He told me that he came one day to see me and he counted more than sixteen tubes going in and out of every orifice. I had renal failure and I was bloated beyond recognition. The new lungs were floating in fluids. I was told that they were too big for my chest cavity and had to be stapled into place. I had no idea what that looked like until three years later when a doctor wanted to show me something in my chest X-ray and I saw the huge staples holding the lungs in place. It was an overwhelming sight.

I still have a lot of questions about that missing period of my life. I would like to know how my husband coped going home every night from the hospital and not certain that he would still meet me in the land of the living when he returned in the morning. I would like to know what it was like for him sleeping on our bed unsure of when or if I would be back to share that bed with him. I still wondered how Ose managed each day going to school being so far away from home. He took his end of year examination not knowing exactly what was going on, knowing fully well that he would get the mother of all summaries from his father. I cannot imagine what it was like for Ehi close enough at home to see his father come in every day from the hospital without any news save; "It is well." Ehi told me later that his dad was calm, very calm. Was that calmness just on the surface and a cover-up for an inner turmoil or was it the peace of God that passes every human understanding that simply engulfed him and garrisoned his heart from every agitating fear? I wanted to know.

I went through the valley of the shadow of death. My life hung on a thread of spider webs with the tensile strength of steel fastened to the Rock of Ages by grace. But for the Lord who was on my side when the enemy rose up against me I would have been swallowed up quick. I found plenty evil to fear in this shadow as I will share in the next chapter. I give praise and glory to God who did not leave me as prey in the teeth of the enemy of our soul. Like a bird escaped from the snare of the fowler, my soul escaped in the valley of the shadow of death.

Not only did God keep me in the hollow of His mighty hands, He kept my husband and my children. He raised up innumerable number of friends and family members to hold us up in prayers. I was overwhelmed when I heard later, the way many friends and even those we did not know personally rose to provide tangible care for my men. They came back home several times from the hospital to meet dinner at the doorstep.

I thank God for the precious gift of life and for the love and care of my dear husband, our sons, families and friends during this period.

#

Somewhere In Between

Stories abound of many people who had dreams and saw visions while in coma. Many people have asked me what it was like to be in coma. It is difficult to explain and recall many of the experiences I had while I was in coma. Some of the visions I had were as vivid as they were frightening. It was a place where the visions I had were as real to me as a physical experience. My coma experience was not a restful one. I was not asleep resting. I was very active, moving from one place to the other. I did not see visions of heaven. But each dream ended in victory as I was delivered from each of the dire situations I found myself in.

I will share in this chapter some of the dreams and visions I had. Some of them were better described as nightmares. They were so real to me that when I came back to the land of the living, I was confused for a while because my perception of reality was distorted by the images and visions I had while I was in limbo.

It was a battle for my life. But not only medically but in the unconscious state I was in. I battled for life in several scenes I saw. Many of the scenes I saw while in coma were scary. They were all about struggling with an unseen force. I saw myself harassed. I saw myself being punished for offenses I did not commit. On one occasion I heard a voice saying to me that I was being punished because of someone else, I do not know who till date. I saw myself being pulled between two forces. Some of the scenes were so vivid that I could recall them with clarity including the distress I felt in the scene.

#

The Carousel: A Disconnect between My Thoughts and Reality.

I opened my eyes to see my husband sitting by my bedside. He wore a green gauze-like gown over his tweed blazer. He turned towards me and said, "I told you I will be here."

"Where am I?" But I did not hear the sound of my voice.
"Where are we?" I tried again.

There was a carousel across the corridor to my bed. There were tables covered with red table cloth with chairs surrounding them to the left side of the corridor behind my husband. The setting was like a tea room opposite the carousel. The room, the hall and the carousel were decorated with vibrant Christmas decorations. I could see snow through the windows and in the background. It was pristine white.

"Where am I?" I tried to move my neck and my hands. It was not possible. It was as if they were tied down, there was something in my neck and inside my throat. Whatever it was, made it difficult for the sound to come out of my throat. My husband did not hear me. He kept asking me what I wanted.

Christmas carol blazed from the carousel and some children sat atop some of the horses. I could not see their faces. But I knew they were there. The carousel made a lot of noise as it went around in circles. I got quite irritated by what I thought was the incessant noise from the carousel, not knowing where I was added to my distress.

In that state of limbo, I thought my husband had told me something went wrong during the transplantation surgery. I had seen him sitting on the grey steps in front of the hospital, each foot rested on different steps. His chin rested on his left hand and his elbow rested on his left knee. He was staring ahead and looked forlorn. The sky over him was blue with scattered clouds. He was there when the doctors came out to tell him they had a problem during the surgery and I had to be evacuated by air to another hospital. He got up and followed them into the hospital.

It appeared to be that my chest had been closed back. I was packed in a box and carried to an airfield. My husband was told that he could not fly in the air-ambulance with me. He had to travel by a commercial plane. He slung a back pack over his shoulder in readiness for the flight. But he told me, he will soon be with me. I have a vague recollection of the inside of the plane. There were some people with me in the plane and it was as if we were in the cargo area. It seemed something happened to my legs while I was packed in the box inside the plane. I recalled being wheeled along a white corridor when we got to the new hospital. And when they opened the box, I saw something wrong with my legs and the doctors were talking about it. I still don't know how I was seeing myself in the box while I was still in the box. It appeared like I was watching a movie but also acting in the movie.

I did not see my husband for a long while after I got to the hospital until when he appeared by my bedside covered in the green gauze-like gown. I had lots of questions for him. I wondered where I could possibly be that it was snowing. I was confused by the Christmas songs and decorations because I knew

I went into the hospital for the surgery in April. I wondered where all the months in-between went.

I wanted to know why he was not there on our 21st wedding anniversary on April 23rd, 2013. I had recalled that on the 22nd I told the nurses that the following day was my wedding anniversary. I heard the nurses telling me "Happy Anniversary" on the morning of the 23rd, but I did not see flowers in the room. That was unusual. My husband always gave me flowers on my birthdays and wedding anniversary. He knew I loved roses. There were no roses and my husband was not there. I was very upset

I got quite restless not being able to get my husband to understand what I wanted from him, at not being able to voice my queries and with the discomfort of not being able to move. I could not move any part of my body save my eyes, which saw all that I thought was taking place. The distress and pain became so much that it set an alarm off, and the bleeping noise of the alarm brought the nurses running into the room.

I heard the nurses ask my husband what had happened. I heard him respond that I got agitated and restless trying to move. The next thing I knew was that I was off again into a dark place. I recall thinking later that I felt I was unduly angry with my husband for not answering my many questions and for not stopping the noisy children on the noisy carousel. Then, I realised I had missed an opportunity of sharing that time with him because it appeared that it had been a long time since I saw him and it would be an even longer time before I would see him again. I promised myself that I will apologise for being mean to him, the next time I saw him.

It was much later that I found out that it was the machines surrounding me that were making all the noise I thought was coming from the carousel and Christmas songs. It had all been a figment of my imagination. . Or at least that was what my mind was telling me was happening. But I did not see those machines that day until much later.

My husband later told me he was right by my side on our wedding anniversary. He told me I had no conversation with the nurses the day before as the doctors were fighting for my life. He also confirmed that there was a day I had opened my eyes. He said that the nurses told him that I had opened my eyes once before he arrived. He told me he had pleaded and prayed that I would open my eyes again while he was there. I did. Whether it was the same day I saw the carousel, I do not know. But there was obviously a disconnect between my mind while in coma and the reality. All that became clear later on.

#

Dream Or Nightmare?

The desert was red hot. The sand dunes were red. The rock face was red. I was covered from head to toe in a black cape with a hood. I did not see my face but I knew it was me. I saw myself tottering along a path on the red hot sand. It was a very rough terrain. It appeared I had escaped from an enclave where I was held captive. I had a vague vision of the enclave, of being made to sit on bare sandy floor and of the atmosphere of intense conflict. There were other people there, but I could not recall their faces. In an instant, I escaped from where I was held captive and began the long weary walk. I somehow got out of that desert. It was as if someone met me on the way and led me out.

In another scene, I found myself in an apartment overlooking a vast fenced wooded area. The apartment was in a multiple level building. Electrical and communication wires crisscrossed the street. There was a familiarity about the environment and yet I knew I had never been there before. It was a strange place. I recalled the setting with vivid accuracy. I knew something weird happened in that apartment and I escaped into the streets but I had no recollection of what happened when I woke up from the coma.

There was yet another scene in which I found myself in a fairly big house. It was an elegantly furnished home of someone whom I seemed to know very well. There was an overwhelming sense of familiarity about the house and its occupants yet I felt I had never been in that particular building before. I was being held against my will. It was in this house that someone appeared to me. It was as if I knew the person well, yet I could not recollect his face. He was the one who told me I was being punished because of someone who in that vision was well known to me. But when I woke up, I could not recall who it was.

There were many other visions where I saw myself constantly being pulled down into a very dark place and then pulled back up into a place full of light. It had an appearance of a cabin where instant photos are taken. I was on a chair pulled down by a force into the dark, and in a flash pulled back up by an opposing force into flashing light.

I still do not understand all the visions I had while I was in coma. But one thing I know for sure is that I was not at rest at all while I was down under. I was like one in a very dark place. The joy I have today is in knowing that even the lawful captives are set free and the prey of the might are delivered (Isaiah 49:24). In all the scenes, God gave me victory. He shone His glorious light into the darkness that enfolded me in each of the scenes and brought me out of them.

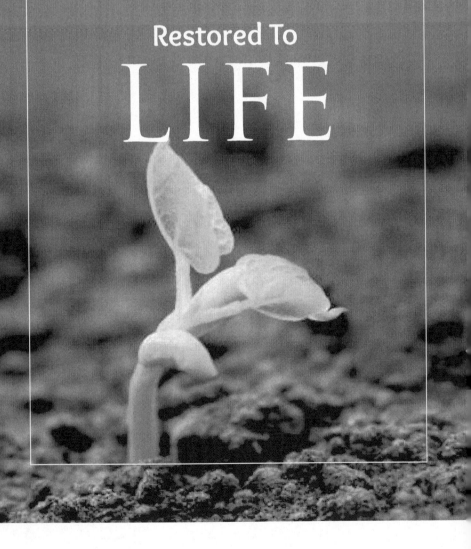

PART FOUR

Restored To
LIFE

Back in the Land of the Living

When I woke up from coma, I felt battle-worn. Tired from an intense struggle between life and death. The visions troubled my spirit as they kept flashing back. I was confused. I had lost track of time. I had no sense of location. I even thought I was in another country away from Switzerland. I did not see my husband for a while and that added to my anxiety and confusion. I wondered why he was not there when I woke up. I could not move my body. I could not speak. I felt lost.

"I will not die but live to declare the goodness of God in the land of the living" (Psalm 118:17) became my constant declaration in my heart during those days after I came back to life and as I was trying to process all that had happened to me. My mind was a battlefield as the enemy brought all sorts of suggestions. I used the Word of God stored up within me to keep my mind from going off track to places I didn't want it to go. Reading the Bible or praying out aloud was impossible at that time. But the word was alive and active in me, and I held fast to it in my mind to override all the suggestions of the enemy assaulting my mind and to forcefully switch my mind back on the right track.

I remembered that the Old Prophet came into the room with a team of doctors shortly after I came back to life. They talked about me as they stood around the bed. I was too delirious to make the effort to follow their discussion in French. But I remembered vividly that the Old Prophet came close to me and said, "You got very strong lungs." There was a firm assertion in his voice. He sounded victorious and yet with a tone of compassion. His tone was certainly different from what I had become familiar with. And that was unnerving.

Day and night became merged together. The clock was ticking but time was meaningless. Pain, distress and overwhelming discomfort were my constant companions. "This has come to pass; this has come to pass" - was the sing-song in my mind. I remember that I was shivering and felt very cold. It took an enormous effort to communicate that to the nurses without speaking, and then they saw my body shaking. They first covered me with a shimmering foil-like fabric. Then they covered me with a canopy that had hot air blowing through it. I became too hot and agitated. I wanted it off. But they did not understand me. It was a wordless communication with blinking and nodding in response to their questions in French. Half the time, I did not understand what they were saying to me.

I watched the nurses grind many drugs together in a mortal, mix it with water and aspirate it into a huge syringe, which must be at least 50mls. I watched them push the content of the syringe through the gastro-nasal tube attached to the side of my face. Many times I almost gagged as the fluid went inside of me, followed by an intense pain in my stomach. I dreaded that pain each time the nurses came to administer the drugs.

I wanted my husband. But it was Bro. O that came. He said my husband was giving a lecture in another country. But that was what I thought he said. He asked me if I wanted to see Ehi. He promised to go and bring him. In my state of confusion, I thought he travelled back to Geneva to bring Ehi, whom he told me was at a basketball camp. I imagined that they arrived and were housed in a hostel above the hospital. It took a long while before he brought Ehi, which further fed my confused conviction that he had travelled somewhere to bring my son.

He did not understand me when I asked for my husband. He did not understand me when I asked where I was. He did not understand me when I asked him to scratch my forehead. It was itchy. I could not lift my hands to scratch it. Every attempt to get people to read my mind through my eyes was abortive. No one seemed to hear the soundless scream from the core of my being.

Finally, my husband came. I was delighted to see him. I wanted to tell him I was sorry about the way I treated him the last time he came. I wanted to ask where he had been. But no words came. He did not understand the questions I thought were clearly written on my face. But I had made up my mind I was not going to get angry the way I did the last time. He sat with me in his green overall and face mask. He held my hand in his gloved hands. I wanted to feel his touch without any barrier but he was required to put on the protective covering. I tried to read his eyes peering at me above the mask. They were deep but unreadable. He spoke to me; his voice was muffled through the mask. I wanted to ask for Ose. I had seen Ehi. Somehow, he started talking about the boys. Then one day, he took off the mask briefly and perched a kiss on the side of my face.

The nurses provided a board with alphabets on it to aid communication. They wanted me to touch the alphabets in response to their questions or communicate what I wanted to say. It was not effective. I was thinking in English. They asked their questions in French. My husband tried it too. I tried to type, "where am I?" I think he finally understood the question because he started talking about the hospital and the surgery.

It was during the times the nurses cleaned me up that I noticed that my toenails were painted with a brilliant red nail polish. The brilliance caught my attention because I usually wear subtle colours. I had a tingling burning sensation around the area above my ankles. A team of doctors came and the nurses removed the blanket covering my legs. They spoke in very quiet tones and left. Soon after, the nurses came back, two of them, with a tray of dressing. The ladies spoke under their breath as they worked on my legs. I could not see what they were doing on the feet because they had lowered that section of the bed below the rest of my body. They bandaged the feet and leg all the way to my knees when they finished.

One morning, the nurses came and told me they were going to sit me up. Fear gripped my heart; "how would it be?" I knew how distressing it was when they turn me thrice a day to clean me up – in the morning, in the afternoon and evening to refresh my body. It was always done by two nurses with such attention to ensure that all the numerous wires and tubes attached to me did not get detached or entangled. They brought a lift. Between, the four of them, they rolled a sheet under me and attached it to the lift. Slowing they lifted me up and turned my body to the left side of the bed. My body felt weightless and limp. My heart was in my mouth as I shot prayers to the heavens. Gently, they lowered the lower part of my body and brought me into a sitting position out of the bed into a padded chair with one of the nurses holding my feet wrapped in heavy bandage. I was sitting again. I was allowed to stay for about half an hour in that position and returned to bed.

I was transferred to another level of intensive care shortly afterward. It was a room encased with glass. Sunlight flooded the room through the window on the right side. I could see the walls of the next building. It was the first time I saw daylight after what seemed to be a very long time. I cannot describe the feeling of liberation it gave me to see natural light again. The nurses' bay was on the left. Nurses and visitors enter the room passing through a cubicle where they must don a protective covering but it had a glass window for someone to look into the room before entering. It was through that window that I saw Sista Iy and my husband coming to see me but they had to be stopped.

One of the nurses had come in earlier in the day to change the urinary catheter. Apparently this has to be changed at a particular frequency. As the day went on, I began to feel very uncomfortable in my tummy. My bladder became painfully full and distended. Something was wrong with the catheter. Urine was not draining from my bladder. For reasons, I could not understand, the bell was hung too far over my head for me to reach and call the nurses. I screamed for attention in agony, no sound came out. I banged the alphabet board on the table with all the strength I could muster. I was frightened and ready to pull out the catheter. The fear of the damage I could cause held me in check. The nurse in the bay heard the banging and came running in just as my husband and Sista Iy entered the cubicle. The nurse saw me writhing in pain holding the base of my abdomen and asked me what was the matter. I pointed to the empty urine bag hanging by the bed. She knew. She pulled her gloves on and examined me. As she began to remove the catheter, she told me to wait for her to grab the bed pan. But I had no control over the bladder as it emptied itself completely on the bed. A wave of relief swept over me. I felt sorry for the poor nurse, pained for having to go through this embarrassment and relief that the bladder was empty, so many emotions at the same time. After the beddings had been changed, my husband and Sista Iy were allowed in. I could not explain to them what had happened in any details, only nodding as they sought to confirm what the nurse had told them.

In all of the distress, pain, discomfort and confusion, I knew God had given me victory. I was like a burning stick snatched out of fire, a branch plucked out of fire (Zechariah 3:2). God rescued me from the jaws of death as He rescued Daniel from the power of the lions (Daniel 6:27). I could not but give praise to God that we hearkened to His voice when He asked us to raise a clarion call for prayers. We had called some of our close friends and our family to stand in the gap for us after my experience with the Old Prophet earlier in this book. I knew people were praying. I felt the force of the prayers as I was pulled out of each scene I saw while I was in coma.

A few days later, my doctors decided that I was stable enough to be transferred back to the hospital in Geneva. On May 15th, 2013, one week after I came out of coma, three men in orange overall came into the room with a stretcher. I was removed from the hospital monitor and attached to the mobile monitor they came with and to a portable oxygen supply. Two men wheeled the stretcher while the third man held the oxygen canister. They placed the bleeping monitor on my laps. My husband could not go with us. He went as far as the lift and he had to leave for Geneva by road. The men took me to the roof of the hospital where a helicopter was waiting. I was strapped down on the floor of the helicopter. The man carrying the oxygen cylinder stayed with me at the back while the other two went into the cockpit. In an instant, the blades started whirling. The noise was almost unbearable. Their ears were covered, mine were not, and we began the trip to the Teaching Hospital in Geneva. We landed on the roof of the hospital and I was transferred to the intensive care unit at the basement of the hospital.

Psalm 54:1-7 summarized my experience especially verse 4. "Surely, God is my helper. He keeps my soul alive." If it were not for God standing by my side when the enemy of my soul rose up against me, then they would have swallowed me up quick (Psalm 124). But thanks be to God Who kept me in His Mighty Hands and snatched me out of the jaws of death. The Lord kept me through the dark night and His Mighty Hands lifted me like an eagle soaring over the stormy blast.

#

They Took My Feet

I am not quite sure the exact time when they broke the news to me. It had to be before I was taken down to the second intensive care unit in the hospital in Lausanne. The images of that day have remained very blurred. I recall that I had noticed the unusually brilliant nail polish and wondered who painted my toenails while I was in coma. I recalled the doctors talking about my feet and the nurses dressing and covering it with bandage. It was when I was transferred back to the hospital in Geneva that the import of what was going on hit me.

The doctors had told me that I received a very good and strong pair of lungs. My husband began to explain the complications that occurred within forty-eight hours of the surgery and why I was placed in medically-induced coma. Then they told me that I had poor blood circulation and insufficient oxygen supply to the extremities—my hands and my feet. The ensuing hypoxia lead to necrosis, that is, death of the tissues in my hands and feet. Apparently, the dead tissue had changed colour and that was what made my nail polish appear more brilliant.

Shocked and stunned, I stared at my husband. He broke the news that the doctors said it would be necessary for them to amputate both my hands and feet. The first thought that crossed my mind was, "what did I come back for?" I could not imagine that after twenty years of coughing and managing life with a chronic respiratory disease, and after all I went through to be given the second chance at life, I had to deal with such a burden.

"How much more can one person take? Have I not suffered enough?" my heart cried out in an indescribable agony. I was beyond tears. My husband told me how the doctors informed him about the situation while I was still in coma. He told me that he refused to take the decision to have my limbs amputated unless I came back to life. He told me how he went back home and he pulled all my shoes into the middle of the bedroom and began to beseech God to let the owner of the shoes to wear them again. Listening to him as he shared that with me touched me at the core of my heart. He is not given to dramas. That gave me a glimpse into depth of the emotions he must have had to deal with while I was in coma and my life hung on a thread spun with a spider's web. I appreciated him the more for not giving up on me or giving me up at a time when all seemed to be over.

My head reeled with questions; "Why? What went wrong? Who was responsible for this?" Not once in all the times the doctors have reeled out the constellation of risks associated with doing a lungs transplant, had anyone mentioned amputation of my limbs.

Dr. G. came to see me. She told me that they have asked all the questions and conducted an audit of the surgery and post-surgical events. They could not find a conclusive explanation for what had happened. Prof. J actually sat with me. He was visibly stunned. I could see the compassion mixed with confusion in his face. No one could offer me any explanation. Soon, I became the object of attraction, every intern and student wanted to see what necrosis looked like. A couple of them even asked me if they could take pictures. It was as if the news spread like a wildfire and they kept coming in their numbers. I was aggrieved and vexed sore in my heart. When an elephant sized problem knocks you down, tiny ants will have the temerity to walk over you. I poured out the bitterness of my soul in silent prayer before God and I complained bitterly to my consultant to put a stop to it. A hood was placed over my feet to cover them. The nurse taking care of the feet kept asking me to take a look at it every morning when she came to dress it and with the same breath she informed me there was no life in the feet. It seemed she was desperate to convince me.

While all of these were going on, my husband had to go on duty travel to Somalia. He could not ask to be relieved from traveling since his head of unit and colleagues in the office were unaware of my medical situation. I wanted him to be with me but I knew he could not because he did not want to involve his work place in our private issues. We had requested the doctors to give us time to make the decision. I think my husband needed that time away to get his head around the decision we had to make. I was hoping and praying for a way out of amputation. Thankfully, Ose had arrived back in Geneva at this time. The young man was by my bedside as long as he was allowed to stay inside the ICU.

As if all I had to gabble with were not bad enough, the attending ICU doctor decided to go on a war path with Dr. G. questioning her every decision. She felt I was stable enough to be moved to the regular ward. I was at this time having several sessions during the day when a speaking valve is connected to the tracheotomy tube, which allowed sounds to come out when I speak. I was still on gastro-nasal feeding. The doctor in charge of the tracheotomy wanted to be sure I would not gag while swallowing before the tracheotomy tubes was removed. I had not been given any fluid or food by mouth. I had been on a long "fast" and I longed for the feel of water in my mouth. They started giving me sugar cube-sized pineapple flavoured ice cube one afternoon to relieve the dryness in my mouth and I wanted more. But I was restricted to just one cube every 3-4 hours. The senior doctors decided that the tracheotomy tube would be kept on until after the amputation. Somehow this did not go down well with this ICU doctor. For reasons best known to her, she wanted me out. She felt I should be handed over to the surgical team, since the only thing keeping me in the ICU was the surgery. And she was a physician. I was an added burden to her workload.

The orthopaedic surgeons mounted more pressure for me to give a go ahead for the amputation to be done right away. They felt it was risky to my lung to delay. I would not be rushed into such a decision. I told them my husband was away on duty travel and we would decide together when he returned. The psychotherapist in the amputation unit came to visit me. She wanted to prepare me for the forthcoming change in my body. She told me I needed to prepare for the change in my body image. I refused to listen to her. I just was not ready to consider that thought. I was hoping against hope that a miracle would happen and I would not have to undergo the amputation.

Two things happened almost simultaneously to bring me to the point of actively dealing with the situation. My quest for a defined answer to my question was preventing me from facing the situation stacked up before me. Dr. G had come to check on me. And I asked her to tell me in all sincerity if there was a way out of having my feet amputated. She looked at me long and hard, and slowly shook her head. I knew her well enough to know that she is as brutally honest as she is fierce in her quest to resolve a situation. She told me I had one option; that I could stay rooted at the spot where I insist I must find an answer to why it happened or I could pick up my life and move on. I was not prepared to hear that from her. But I knew she told me the hard truth I needed to hear.

Then my husband sent me a message from Somalia. He said, God has promised to give me the 'feet of grace' that would take me to places my natural feet would not have taken me. That word of hope and assurance came through our family friend, Bro. G., who was also on the same mission in Somalia with my husband. The word offered me hope even though I felt no tangible comfort at that point in time. Life was returning to my hands at this time but not to my feet.

When my husband came back two days later, we knew that we had no choice but to submit to the amputation. We called our sons in and told them that I would have to undergo the amputation of my feet. We all wept together as we processed in our mind the gravity of the decision we made. The nurse on duty put the screen around us to give us some privacy and requested the rest of the team to stay away for a while from my bed. When we felt ready to face the doctors, we called them in and told them they could go ahead with the amputation. That day was May 28th, 2013. It is a day I am not likely to forget in a long time.

I made two requests to the doctors after the decision was made that the surgery would take place on Friday, May 31st. I asked if I could be allowed to stand up on the feet for one last time. The answer was a firm negative. It was not possible. I began to recall the last time I stood on my feet. It was on Saturday, April 13th, when I was asked to undress in readiness to go to the theatre for the lungs transplant. I stood up from the bed so that my husband could help me remove my trousers. I remembered that I placed my hands on his shoulder as he bent down to lift up my feet to remove the trousers. I never knew then that was the last time I would be standing on my natural feet.

Then I made my second request. I asked if I could be taken out of the ICU to the terrace on top of the unit. I wanted to feel the warmth of the sun and the gentle touch of the breeze one time before my body is transformed. The initial answer was negative. No one would permit that nor would any of the nurses be willing to accompany me with all the gadgets. Eventually, Dr. G decided that she would pursue it. She sought the approval of the Chief of the Intensive Care Unit presenting the whole picture. I needed to be in a good mental state before going in for the life-transforming surgery. The Chief agreed only if one nurse would volunteer to take me out. Simply put, no one was under obligation to take such a risk. Eventually one of the nurses agreed. They fixed the speaking valve. I was lifted into a wheelchair, taken off the monitor with only the monitor for oxygen saturation attached to my finger. I was connected to a mobile oxygen bottle and covered from neck down with a light blue blanket. I wore a face mask until we got outside and with my husband. we began the trip to the roof of the unit. The sun was setting but it was still warm. I felt it on my forehead. The nurse positioned me in a secluded part of the garden where there was no one and we could have some privacy. She went to sit away from us but kept me in sight while giving my husband and I sometime alone.

We called our parents. We could not get through to my parents-in-law at that time. I spoke first to my father and my mother. They knew I had the transplant. They knew I had been in the

ICU but that was all the information we released to them. It was the first time they were hearing my voice in almost two months. The 15 minutes allowed went too fast but God gave us the opportunity for me to speak with my parents-in-law when I got back into the ICU just before the speaking valve was removed. I was grateful for the touch of the wind. I was grateful for the warmth of the sun. They reminded me that God is alive in heaven. They reminded me that I am still alive and in the land of the living. The future may look dim but I will declare the goodness of God in the land of the living. There is a purpose for all of these even if I could not see it. That was the day before my feet were removed. It was Thursday, May 30th, 2013.

That night one of the attending surgeons came to mark and measure my legs. He signed my thighs with iridescent pen. He explained what would happen the following day. They would come for me at 6:00am. That was all I heard. Everything else blew over my head. I tried to keep my mind on one track; I am alive! I told myself God who knows it all knows it best. I had no idea how I would cope with life when I come out of the theatre the following day. Morning came too fast. As on time as the Swiss clock, they were there with the gulley to wheel me into the theatre again for a life-transforming surgery in less than two months since I was last there for a life-giving surgery.

I was given an epidural anaesthesia. I braced myself for sleep after they gave me medications to calm my nerves and put me in a mild sleep. I heard whirring sounds. I heard voices. I opened my eyes and I saw hooks hanging overhead. After a while, they woke me up and told me the surgery was over. I knew what that meant; my legs had been cut off from below the knee. I had been transformed from full bodied individual to a bilateral amputee.

Life was not going to be the same as before again. Something massive had changed.

They wheeled me out of the theatre and back into the ICU. My husband was waiting along the corridor to receive me. He took my hand and I looked at him with tears rolling down the side of my head, "they took my legs" that was all I could say. My legs were gone. "It will be alright" was his only response.

He sat by my bedside for the rest of the day holding my hand as I drifted in and out of sleep. Sensation began to return to my left leg as the anaesthesia wore away, and with it came pain. The nurses told me to administer morphine as needed by pushing the red button on the pump kept by my side. But I was scared because there was no sensation in my right leg. Then the enemy began to torture me with "what ifs" that I could not find immediate answers for. I knew then again; I must not allow his suggestions to take root in my heart. I had come a long way and had a long journey ahead. I would not entertain any suggestion that I may not regain sensations in my right leg or what is left of it. My husband explained what could have happened while the epidural was being injected and that it was not a strange thing. It took several more hours before I could feel the right leg.

One chapter of my life was closed and another was set to begin. All I could say to myself was that He who knows the future knows what the future holds for me. He holds my future in His hands. He is obligated because of His unfailing love to see me through the next phase of my life.

#

The Breath of Joy

The day was Sunday, June 2nd, 2013, two days after the amputation of my limbs. My husband had sent me a text as they left home for church. He and the boys were coming after church. I longed for their visit. Hospital is a lonely place to be and I was in a very lonely place emotionally. I was simply spent and empty. I waited and waited. Service should have been over by 12:30pm. I gave them an extra hour to get to the hospital but the hour passed and they had not showed up. It was First Sunday of the month and a Thanksgiving service. They would certainly be longer than usual because of the birthday celebrations. But I was silently wishing they would not stay for any of the post-service activities and just come straight to me.

They did stay. It was Aunty Funke's birthday. She is one of those in the forefront praying for us. I could not deny them sharing the joy of the day with her. I was holding a me and myself conference in my heart as I remembered why they would be late coming to the hospital. How often had they had to come to the hospital straight from the church in the past? I could not count even if I tried. "Give them a break. Let them have life." I admonished myself.

A short while later they appeared at the door, all three of them with their face masks on. I was thrilled. I was not going to complain about the pain in my left or discomfort of moving on the bed with the blue soft cast around both legs. I wanted us to have a family time together. I was making some progress with the use of my hands as life and functionality was being restored. I had done some scribbling earlier in the day. I wanted to share that with them.

They talked about the service and a bunch of other things. Then one of the nurses walked up to my bed and said she was going to take off the nasal cannula that supplied the oxygen to me. I was taken aback. "Pour quoi?" I asked her why in French. She told me she had stopped the flow of the oxygen for the past two hours and the saturation had remained stable at 99%.

I could not believe that after six years of continuous dependence on supplemental oxygen, I was breathing on my own without any external support. She switched off the ventilator and removed the oxygen tube, I took a deep breath on my own and oxygen saturation remained stable. It was pure joy. My heart sang for joy; it was like a dream—when the Lord turned away our captivity we were like them that dream. Then my mouth was filled with laughter and my tongue with singing... (Psalm. 126: 1,2). My husband and my sons rejoiced with me. I was happy they were there when it happened. I began to hum the chorus

> *God, You are so good,*
> *God, You are kind*
> *God, You are wonderful*
> *My God, You are excellent*

That singular event was a turning point. It took my focus off the amputation and took the sting out of the pain of the moment. We were totally focused on the strange and awesome work the Lord had done. We recalled how many times we had had close shaves with the oxygen finishing in the past when we were out of the house. And here was I breathing without fear or panic. I was not breathless. It could only have been God. My husband and sons left for home with a smile on their faces and I knew their hearts were full of joy. For the first time, I was not upset that they were leaving. I was too happy and full of joy, praising God from the depth of my heart.

Oh! I worship the Lord. My soul magnifies His Holy name. I will sing psalms and shout for joy. God has been good to me and my family. He broke the gates of brass and cut the bar of iron asunder. The shackles are broken and I am set free. God is worthy of my adoration. I will prostrate before Him when I get the chance and give Him thanks.

Many see me now and are amazed, some even burst into tears of joy especially those who knew where I was coming from and what happened post-surgery. They are excited and overjoyed when they see me breathing on my own, no tubes attached and talking with fullness of life; it is overwhelming even for me! I am a wonder unto many, even to my doctors, nurses, care givers and therapists. Every day God gives me brand new testimonies and reasons to give praise to Him.

I thank God for the grace He has given me to go through this period and to prepare me for the next phase. My hospital stay had been lengthened by the complications I suffered after the first surgery. The next phase requires a lot of rehabilitation. The Lord Who brought me this far does not do half measures. As He promised, He will restore my health and heal my wounds. He will surely perfect all that concerns me.

> **I was not ready to bear my soul to someone who does not share my faith in God and who would not bring the mind of God to me at such a time.**

#

Rough Road to Rehabilitation

A Gnawing Question

"What has the lungs got to do with legs?"

That was the question on the lips of the nurses who lined the corridor as I was wheeled into the Medical Ward on June 5th, 2013. This was the ward where I had been a regular visitor as a patient for the past ten years. I knew every single nurse on the ward. I had formed a great relationship with them. They all knew me very well. Tears rolled down their faces. I kept a straight face.

———— ✳✳ ————

Hope is my anti-depressant. This was strictly between me and God.

———— ✳✳ ————

My seven weeks and three days' sojourn in the Intensive Care Units of the two hospitals were over and the lungs transplantation was successful.

It was five days after my legs were amputated below the knees.

When the nurses asked, "what has the lungs got to do with legs?" They echoed the questions in my heart.

Though God had told us that He would give me the 'feet of grace' that would take me to places my natural feet could not take me, and though I knew Him as the God who makes promises and fulfils them, at that point in time, that promise did not make any sense to me. I could not get my head around how chronic respiratory diseases could have resulted in the amputation of my feet. I did not see that coming. There was no forewarning of this anywhere in my memory and believe me, I searched.

The nurses asked me, "Are you angry?" Who was I to be angry with? I was not given a culprit to be angry with? The nurses who have become my friends wanted me to talk about the pain, anger and disappointment they expected that I must be feeling.

"You have a right to be angry."

> **It is at such times that you know you have to make an active and deliberate decision to tap into the grace of God that is readily available and sufficient sustain you.**

"With whom?" I queried in my heart, staring blankly over the shoulders of the Psychiatrist and her assistant standing by my bedside at the light grey wall behind them. They came to visit me after the nurses could not get me to talk about the anger and resentment they thought I was storing up inside of me.

The doctors had done the audit. Nobody could explain what went wrong. There was no negligence reported or indicated. So who was I supposed to be angry with? God? I mused, still not saying a word.

"It is important to express your emotions. You can grieve about this. Talk to us." The Psychiatrist cajoled me.

"I don't have anything to say." I looked straight at her and smiled. "I have asked all the questions I can ask the doctors about this."

They told me it was alright to be angry or to cry if I felt like doing so. They wanted me to be willing to talk about how I was feeling about the situation—a case of being dealt with a bad hand, anyone would say. After all, there are many logical reasons to be angry, after twenty years of living with a chronic and debilitating respiratory disease, with my life literally hanging on a thread spun with spider webs during the latter seven years, why should I have to go through another calamity when I just got a miraculous victory over the respiratory problem? I certainly had every right to throw mega fits of anger. But I did not. What is the point of talking with them, I wondered? What could they do for me? Do they have answers to my questions? What comfort could they offer me? I was not ready to bear my soul to someone who does not share my faith in God and who would not bring the mind of God to me at such a time.

> I will not be ashamed of my body. If I am not ashamed of me, then nobody can make me feel ashamed of my body. I will not play the victim. I will not, by the grace of God, be a subject of pity.

> Grace enabled me to latch on the word of assurance God gave me a few days before the amputation - He has given me the Feet of Grace.

"I'm Okay. I am taking one day at a time." I told her. They went on again about my need to talk. They thought I was in denial. I even found out later that they put me on a low dose of anti-depressant medication. They thought because I wasn't talking to them, I was depressed and not dealing with the issue. They asked the nurse who had known me the longest during my ten years of frequent sojourn on that ward to come and talk to me.

She tried. And I could see that she was visibly upset that I was not willing to open up to her. So I said to her, "*J'ai décidé depuis longtemps que je ne jamais renouncer l'espoir. Mon espoir est à mon Dieu.*" I had made up my mind a long time ago that I will never give up on hope, and I was not going to start now. My hope is in God alone. It was on that note that she left me alone.

I repeated the same to the Psychiatrist when she came back to see me, and begged her to stop the medication. I told her I did not need it. Hope is my anti-depressant. This was strictly between me and God. The doctors could not answer the questions running all over my head. I was in deep pain, and it was not a physical pain. I was even angry for a while and I did not know where to direct my anger. But God surely understood where I was coming from when I cried out to Him in the dead of the night when there was not one near to hear my cry.

> It was helpful and uplifting for us to do this together as a family. I appreciated my husband and sons even the more that they did not leave me to walk this path alone but they held my hands and walked the path along my side.

For many days after the amputation, I refused to look at the stumps. When the nurses asked me if I wanted to see them during the dressing of the stumps, my response was an emphatic "No!" and I turned away my face. The wounds healed with such an amazing rapidity that I could not help but notice the joy lighting up the face of the nurse when she looked up and said, "they are healing well. It is remarkable."

Finally, I looked. First at the space where the rest of my legs and feet should have been. Then at the stumps. The skin was very dry and peeling off in big chunks. It required that we applied a special lotion every night before putting a light gauze stocking and bandage over them. My husband offered to do it when the nurse came in the night to apply the lotion. Then the following nights, my sons took turns to apply the lotion and bandage the stumps before leaving the hospital to go back home. They did not show any ackwardness touching the stumps. It was a huge deposit on my self-esteem account. My husband and sons were not ashamed to touch my stumps—that was huge for me.

I finally got myself to hold my stumps. I cradled them in my hands. I looked at what was and is left of my legs. Tears laced my eyes. I blinked them away. "I will not cry," I told myself. I refused to sorrow over the situation.

Nothing prepares anyone for such a situation. Not once in my almost 47 years before that day, did I ever imagine I could be at that phase of life with missing limbs. A fellow amputee told me that it was worse to wake up and find your limb gone. I had the opportunity to process the amputation before it happened. For that, I appreciated my husband the more for not taking the decision about the amputation while I was still in coma. It is at such times that you know you have to make an active and deliberate decision to tap into the grace of God that is readily available and sufficient sustain you.

> **Then God spoke to my heart, "sing praises."**

Graham Kendrick's song, "*To You, O Lord I lift up my soul*" from Psalm 25 floated back into my spirit. The lyrics ministered to me:

No one whose hope is You will ever be put to shame.
That's why my eyes are on You O Lord
Surround me, defend me
O how I need You
To You O Lord I lift up my soul

My hope is in God. I cannot be put to shame because God will defend me and surround me with His love and mercy. I will not be ashamed of my body. If I am not ashamed of me, then nobody can make me feel ashamed of my body. I will not play the victim. I will not, by the grace of God, be a subject of pity. If I keep my head and my spirit high, no one will be able to pity me or my situation. I spoke these words to myself over and over again until they took root in my heart.

I could not afford to behave like one without hope. Because of all I had been through over the past years, I knew that to be alive at that point in time and breathing without any support or effort in itself is a miracle and a precious gift. Grace kept directing and leading me to focus on that miracle. That became the focus of my attention. It became my *raison d'etre* to give thanks and praise to God amid the continuing storm. Grace enabled me to latch on the word of assurance God gave me a few days before the amputation - He has given me the Feet of Grace.

The psychotherapist working with amputees came and sat with me several afternoons. She had tried to talk to me before the amputation. I was not ready to listen to what she had to say then. And I refused to read the information materials. She was resilient. She did not push me to talk. She just wanted me to know that I have to deal with the change in my body image.

Let me note here, if you are ever with someone who has lost a limb, please don't ever tell the person that there are many people living with missing limbs and doing great, some are even running and are champions! Yes, you are right but "Why do I have to be one of them?" was my reaction. That is not what an amputee wants to hear, certainly not at the beginning when the person has to adjust emotionally to a body with conspicuously missing parts.

This lady waited until I was ready to talk about the change in my body. Then she supported me and my family to get all the information we needed to cope with our new definition of normal. Then, they arranged for us to watch a video of people living with amputation. We watched it as a family there in the hospital. We were able to ask more questions. It was helpful and uplifting for us to do this together as a family. I appreciated my husband and sons even the more that they did not leave me to walk this path alone but they held my hands and walked the path along my side.

#

To Walk Again

Miraculously, my stumps healed within two weeks after the surgery. The surgeons were stunned when they examined the wound. They kept calling other doctors to come and see. It was the first time in that hospital that they would have an amputation and they did not have to go back to the theatre at least one more time because of infections or heamatoma, which is the collection of blood in the wounds. They were happy for me. But I was numb and quiet. I still didn't get the situation. I had not been able to hold the stumps at that time. I even looked away from them.

My agonising desire was to be able to swing my legs out of my bed and stand up right. I remembered that morning in June 2013; the desire to stand and walk was so overwhelming that my heart throbbed with such indescribable pain that the streaming tears burnt my cheeks. I fixed my gaze on the wide ceiling of my hospital room and let the tears flow.

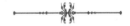

I knew I had to make a choice. I could be happy and joyful that I was finally standing again, or I could be sad and morose that I am never going to have painted toenails or wear dainty slippers again. The choice was mine and mine alone.

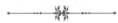

To walk again, just to be able to stand upright and walk again, I never knew that a time would come in my life that this would be the earnest fervent cry of my heart. The years of jogging and competitive running flashed back. And my heart ached with the desire; to stand up and walk again. Then God spoke to my heart, "Sing praises." I thought my mind was playing a trick on me. "Sing praises."

"Sing praises?" Really?" It took me a while before I yielded to the voice nudging me to sing praises. I began to sing softly under my breath some songs of praise. The more I sang the more the heavy cloud of grief hanging over me lifted, and the louder I sang, until God gave me a brand new song. It was a song that came fresh into my heart and I formed the lyrics as I sang. Before I knew it I was singing a new song to the Lord and He lifted the dark clouds, my spirit was lift. I was still singing when the nurses came in. They smiled. They had always known me to sing during my hospital stay. I guess they were happy to hear me singing again that morning.

> But for one brief moment, I took my eyes off the prosthesis, and I looked up; "I am standing. I am actually standing."

I knew first-hand, what life must be like for amputees who may never have the chance to walk again. The tag line for the yet-to-be conceived foundation fell like a seed on fertile ground that morning – that all may walk again.

The normal waiting period before starting the process of making the prostheses was six months. Rather than waiting for this period, my doctors decided to initiate the process immediately since my stumps had healed miraculously very fast. There was no need to wait any longer, they opined. I went for the casting and they created the mould that would become the cup of the prostheses.

We had a long argument about the kind of shoes and the height of heels I could wear. I struggled with my emotions as the physiotherapist told me that my new feet were to be customized to a fixed angle which will allow me to wear flat shoes not more than 2cm high. They strongly recommended snickers for security as it would clad the entire foot and help me to maintain my balance.

"What! Only one type of shoes every day?" My voice was several decibels higher than normal. My eyes must have been flashing because I was not amused in the least. "That is not possible. I can't wear sneakers seven days of the week!" I stated with an undeniable emphasis like a five-year-old denied a delight. If I had a foot I would have stamped it on the ground. They explained to me why I needed to wear shoes with sturdy and broad heels. "What on earth was I to do with all the shoes I have in varying shapes and heights?"

> She said, "No one expects you to be a super-Christian. It is okay to cry. You can approach God and tell Him how you feel. You can ask Him why, and you can pour out your heart to Him."

"It is for your safety. You have to maintain your balance. You must not fall."

I wouldn't hear of it. I walk like a duck in flats. And by the way, "who wears snickers all day long every day, even with Iro and Buba or Ankara long skirts?" I am a Yoruba woman. I wear Nigerian and African outfits. I am proudly African. I don't wear only pants and jeans. I simply refused to accept only sneakers as an option, not even in the name of safety and security. They refused to accept my all low-heeled shoes

> I didn't want anyone to feel sorry for me. This was strictly between me and God, between a daughter and her Father!

because they were not completely covered, and my feet could slip out of them. Finally, they agreed to the pair of shoes I used on field trips and visits to communities when I was working with UNICEF in Cairo. The shoes were completely covered in front with a zipper but 3cm high.

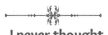

I never thought that putting one foot in front of the other could be such a challenging task. By the end of that week, I was able to walk the length of the parallel bars, a distance of three metres.

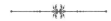

The moulding was done. The cup was made with hard plastic material. We had agreed on the arch of the feet. The day I was to have my first fitting with the provisional prostheses finally came. But none of the discussions we had with the psychotherapist prepared me for that day.

My stumps had to be bandaged tightly in the morning to reduce the volume. That was why I was sitting in a waiting room across the workshop for the volume of the stumps to go down well enough for me to try on the provisional prostheses. It was summer, the time to adorn dainty slippers and reveal painted toenails. That summer was no exception. It had been a parade of slippers and painted toenails. That was my first summer without painted toenails and dainty slippers.

As I sat on my wheelchair waiting, it was as if every lady in the hospital had been summoned to parade their dainty slippers and their beautifully manicured painted toenails in front of me. One after the other, as they cat-walked the corridor in an orchestrated parade, their dainty slippers and painted toenails taunted me. "You ain't gonna do this again" they screamed at me.

I felt as if the enemy was flashing in my face what I had lost and would not be able to do again. Pain and grief welled up from within me. My slippers at home flashed before my sight. I fought back the hot tears stinging my eye lids. I blinked them off. I will not cry here. No, I will not!

It was during the long dreary and sometimes painful journey of rehabilitation and learning to walk again that the idea to establish the Feet of Grace Foundation was conceived.

The technician came to check on me. It was time to try on the prostheses made for me. The bandages around the stumps were removed. When they presented to me the prostheses with yellow cup, metal stems attached to the light "oyinbo" skin covered feet in my zip-up shoes, my heart revolted against it. I wished someone had told me then that what was presented to me was provisional. They would have saved me weeks of distress. I simply could not imagine that was what I would be wearing for the rest of my life. Thinking it was the final product, with great distress, I put on the protective iceross liner, then layered on the socks. They slipped the plastic cups on top of the prosthesis over my stumps, and rolled up the elastic band that held the socket over my thighs.

The technicians and physiotherapists helped me to put on the prosthesis, which we named the "feet of grace." They wheeled me in front of two parallel bars. It was time to get off my butt. After months of laying on the bed, then oscillating between the bed and the wheelchair; it was finally time for me to rise up and stand again for the first time on the "feet of grace." The physiotherapists stood by my sides and gently lifted me up from the wheelchair to stand on the "feet of grace."

I was standing. I was really standing upright. It felt strange. It had been a long time I stood up straight. They placed my hands on the parallel bars. I stood erect between the bars. I looked down at the "feet of grace" - the yellow plastic cup, the metal rod connecting the cup to the feet in the black zip-up pumps we finally settled for.

No dainty slippers. No painted toenails. But I was standing again.

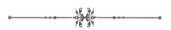

I bless God for every single step I took with those legs. I blessed Him for all the opportunities He gave me to go places with them. I thank God for the time I had with them. They have fulfilled their assignment and have gone home ahead of me. The season of painted toenails and dainty slippers was over. It was great fun while it lasted.

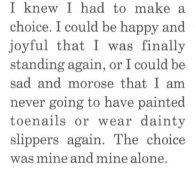

I knew I had to make a choice. I could be happy and joyful that I was finally standing again, or I could be sad and morose that I am never going to have painted toenails or wear dainty slippers again. The choice was mine and mine alone.

At that point in time, I was not thinking about choices. All I was seeing were the challenges of life as an amputee. But for one brief moment, I took my eyes off the prosthesis, and I looked up; "I am standing. I am actually standing."

At first I wobbled on the "feet of grace" and the ladies (my physiotherapists) looped their arms behind me. Then I straightened my body, pulled my frail shoulders up and my bony chest out. I almost missed the opportunity to be grateful for that moment. I almost allowed the sight of the prosthesis to mar the joy of being able to stand.

The day was June 30th, 2013. That day will remain etched in my memory. It was exactly one month after the amputation. And it was a miracle to be trying out a prosthetic limb so soon. For most people, it takes up to six months before starting the process of ambulation. So I guess this unusual feat, never heard off before in that hospital, should give me many reasons to be joyful and dancing on my wheelchair after my first standing session.

> **So I wear my Feet of Grace with grace and head lifted high to the glory of God.**

I thought so too.

But when I got to back to my room, flashes of painted toenails and, dainty slippers oscillated with flashes of plastic cup, metal stem and "oyinbo" skin-coloured feet in black zip-up shoes. I bowed my head on the table in front of me, frail shoulders arched over the table trembled as an indescribable pain seared my heart. I wept.

It was in that state, my dear SistaFriend called me from Nigeria. I poured my heart out to her. She said, "No one expects you to be a super-Christian. It is okay to cry. You can approach God and tell Him how you feel. You can ask Him why, and you can pour out your heart to Him."

I had been trying to be stoic. I thought I could take it in my stride. After all, I am alive. But I had to be honest with God with my feelings. I had to be honest that I was angry and I did not like what had happened to me. I had to be honest that I wanted to know the "why" behind after all I had been through; why I had to go through another complication in my life.

I wept before the Lord. I poured out my pain, my anger and my questions to God. I did it when I was alone. I did not want the pity of anyone. I didn't want the nurses to see me and crowd around me. I didn't want anyone to feel sorry for me. This was strictly between me and God, between a daughter and her Father!

He wrapped His arms around me and held me close to His chest. His breath enveloped me. He spoke His peace to my heart. He gave me an assurance that there is purpose in all of these.

An understanding of God as a God of purpose, Who is not haphazard in His dealing became a life-saver for me at this time. With the encouragement of my husband, sons and friends, I began to focus on the victory God gave us through the valley of the shadow of death. God gave me the precious gift of grace to regain my cheerfulness, to keep my smile on come what may, and stay focused on the goal—to walk again.

The following day, I was back at the workshop. We repeated the process. But on this day, I took my first step forward. It was with great difficulty and pain. I barely lifted the foot off the ground, and move my leg all the way up from my hips to push the foot forward, then I moved the second one. They began to teach me how to move my legs, to land on my heel and roll forward. I learnt there is a technique for walking with prosthesis as a bilateral amputee so I do not hurt my back. I took a few more steps forward. I never thought that putting one foot in front of the other could be such a challenging task. By the end of that week, I was able to walk the length of the parallel bars, a distance of three metres.

The following week, I began to use the walker, which provided me with support while walking; there was only one physiotherapist with me. They took me from the workshop on the fifth floor to the physiotherapy department on the seventh floor. The corridor was marked by metres. There were red and white cones on the floor. There was also an elevated platform with railings on its sides, both ends were slopes. It was here I learnt how to walk up an elevation. The incline was about 30 degrees. That required another style so that I do not fall backwards or forward because of the rigid ankle. It was on that corridor that I walked my first 20 metres, then 60 and 100 metres.

The more I thought of all the books I had waiting to be written, the more determined I got about practicing how to write again.

I was then transferred to the Rehabilitation Home at Beau Sejour, which was more equipped with preparing amputees for an autonomous life out of the hospital. I was taught how to take care of myself in the bathroom, transferring from the wheelchair to the bed, toilet and bath benches without support. I learnt to climb the stairs. The first time I thought I could not lift my feet that high and push forward, I did. And I climbed ten steps by the end of my first week in the Home. One day, I walked 200 metres.

They allowed me to begin to use the crutches. In the big warehouse-like room attached to the Home, they created several scenes of day-to-day life with props there. I was taught how to enter a car, climb into the bus and cross the road among other activities.

It was during the long dreary and sometimes painful journey of rehabilitation and learning to walk again that the idea to establish the Feet of Grace Foundation was conceived. I pondered on how amputees in Nigeria were coping considering the peculiarity of the environment. I wondered what kind of support systems were available to them. How do they afford the huge cost of prosthetic limbs? Those questions fuelled my desire to know more and to seek what I could do.

My new feet were customized for the zip-up black shoes. This was my only pair of shoes for months. Much later, we went to shops with measuring tape until my husband found me broad-heeled shoes with the same height and a bit dressier. I knew I had to let go of my shoes. It would be a torture to keep them and moan over them when they could be a blessing to others. When I got back home from the hospital, I brought all my shoes out. I had a farewell party with them. I gave thanks to God for the joy of having them and asked God to make them a blessing to all those who would wear them for me. We bagged the shoes, many of them with their bags, and with joy and peace in my heart, I released them to go to my friends. I pleaded with a number of them to wear them for me. But I could not let go of my oldest pair of shoes—my first set of purple shoes. That remains a memento of the days of my passion for shoes.

Later on, I went in search of photographs of my legs, only to find that most of the time, my legs were covered in long skirts, trousers and wrappers. Those in which I was wearing short skirts were not showing my legs or painted toenails. Who goes out of their way to take photographs of their legs and painted toenails? Later, I found the photograph taken at my first son's high school graduation. It turned out to be the best picture of my old legs. It was a gift from God. He knew I needed to see those legs again in their former glory. The last time I saw them as such was when I stood up and changed into the theatre gown before my lungs transplantation. It was also the last time I stood on them.

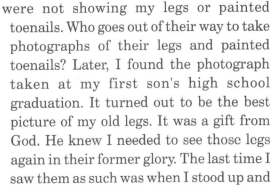

Because my nails were still connected to a source of life, they experienced a turnaround for good and restoration.

I perused every detail of my legs in the picture. But rather than be sorrowful, my heart lifted with joy. I bless God for every single step I took with those legs. I blessed Him for all the opportunities He gave me to go places with them. I thank God for the time I had with them. They have fulfilled their assignment and have gone home ahead of me. The season of painted toenails and dainty slippers was over. It was great fun while it lasted. Like a dear sister wrote to me, there await me a glorious pair of legs when I get to heaven.

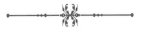

But God did not create us to be stagnant, static or to remain on the same spot. God created us to be active. He created us for growth and for increase. We must resolve to move beyond the dark season. But to do so, we must remain vitally connected to the source of life.

For the rest of my stay here on

earth, God has provided me with the Feet of Grace that will take me to places beyond my imagination and to where my natural feet could not have taken me, just as He promised. He has given me the tools I need to fulfil my assignment and the purpose for which He called me. So I wear my 'Feet of Grace' with grace and head lifted high to the glory of God.

The grace of God is always abundantly available and sufficient for every storm, for every difficult situation and every challenging circumstance that we go through in life. But we have to choose to lay hold of it as if our next breath depends on it.

Andrea Crouch's song "Through It All" was an elixir for my soul during that season.

> I've had many tears and sorrows,
> I've had questions for tomorrow,
> there's been times I didn't know right from wrong.
> But in every situation,
> God gave me blessed consolation,
> that my trials come to only make me strong.
>
> I thank God for the mountains,
> and I thank Him for the valleys,
> I thank Him for the storms He brought me through.
> For if I'd never had a problem,
> I wouldn't know God could solve them,
> I'd never know what faith in God could do

Though, I still cannot wake up in the morning, swing my legs out of bed and walk into the bathroom. But I am walking again, not just a short distance, I can walk kilometres. I can take long strides. I can fast walk. May be someday, I will even do a half-marathon. It was that longing to walk again that sparked the idea of establishing a Foundation that can help and support amputees to stand up and walk again. Feet of Grace Foundation is the manifestation of that dream. In "**Beyond The Storm**" I will describe how the impact of God's power to turn situations around for good is being made evident, not only in my life but also in the lives of many who would not have had the opportunity to walk again. My pain has become the gain for many and God gets all the glory.

#

My Hands Restored

My hands also suffered from insufficient blood and oxygen supply. I noticed that they had changed colour and were darker. There were several spots of dead tissues on my fingers. Miraculously, life began to return to my hands. My doctors determined that they would make good recovery. At the beginning, the hands trembled violently making it difficult to hold things but I began to make the effort to feed myself. The nurses gave me straws for my drinks and a cup with a spout for my tea so that I do not pour the hot tea on myself while my hands were trembling. I began to learn to write again. At first, it was worse than a chicken scrawl. I could not hold my hands steady enough to write legibly but I persisted and made improvement every passing day. Sometimes it took almost 15 minutes to type a short sentence of a text message. That was very frustrating. My fingers kept pressing several keys at the same time because I could not hold them steady. I had so much in my head I wanted to write down I was almost bursting with the gush like a dammed swollen river. Writing had been a lifeline for me in times of great distress. It was a channel through which I poured out my heart. I was scared that I would not be able to write again. The more I thought of all the books I had waiting to be written, the more determined I got about practicing how to write again.

As the dead tissues were excavated from my fingers, I developed sores around the fingers I had to spend several months attending the surgical clinic to ensure that there was no dead tissue retained. This meant, on some occasions they had to go very deep into the flesh to remove the dead cells. I noticed changes on my finger nails. They were discoloured, some were deformed, a few just fell off and some had what looks like blood clot under the nail. There was also a dark band and indentation across the nails. I had bandages over three fingers at the same time to preserve the soft tissues after the nails fell off.

As my fingers became re-oxygenated, they recovered and a new season of refreshing came upon the nails. Subsequently, I observed that as the nails grew, the dark bands moved up and after sometime, the part of the nail above the dark bands literally separated along the line above the bands and in some cases a part of it was still attached to the nail bed, causing a lot of discomfort.

Each time I look at my nails during the dark season of adversity they experienced, I remember an incidence a few years back while I was working in Tamale, Ghana. My second son, Ehi, was five years old and had been ill on and off for a while. So, I took him with me on a trip from Tamale to Accra, where I was scheduled to attend a series of meetings at the Country office, and to see the UN staff doctor for a check-up. After the consultation with the doctor, I left him in the care of my colleague while I attended my meetings. My colleague gave Ehi sheets of paper to draw on and colour to keep him occupied. He sketched what appeared to be long and tapering objects and coloured the tips red. When asked what he had drawn, Ehi promptly responded, "Mummy's fingers and long nails." Well, I took good care of my fingers and kept well-manicured nails. His aggravation was that I kept my nails long while I insisted on having his nails cut. I even had friends tell me that I could be a nail/finger model because my hands, fingers and nails were kept in immaculate condition. I wondered during the dry season if they would ever recover and be restored to their previous state.

Despite the extremely difficult circumstances my nails were subjected to, they struggled to grow again because the living part at the base of the nail was still active. The dark bands eventually reached the tip of my fingers and I could cut them off. It has now become a figment of my memory that they once experienced a season of darkness. All but two of the fingers have the fingers nails restored to their normal shape. The remaining two are still disfigured, a reminder of what I have been through. Because my nails were still connected to a source of life, they experienced a turnaround for good and restoration.

I had several months of therapy to help restore full functionality to my hands. Now I am writing and typing, and doing everything I use to do before without any difficulty.

At one time or the other, we are visited with seasons of darkness and vicissitudes, which forms dark bands across the landscape of our lives. These are seasons of pain, hurt, disappointment, rejection and grief. They are seasons when the fulfilment of our dreams and desires look bleak. Seasons when we appear to be rooted to the same spot or going around the same mountain for so long and our breakthrough seems not forthcoming. We experience seasons when we are treated unfairly or unjustly, and periods of trials and tests, of insufficiency and lack, and of troubles – spiritual, physical and emotional.

But God did not create us to be stagnant, static or to remain on the same spot. God created us to be active. He created us for growth and for increase. We must resolve to move beyond the dark season. But to do so, we must remain vitally connected to the source of life. The evidence of life is growth and movement.

God has equipped us with the capability to move forward and to move on beyond the season of adversity.

My hands are not only writing again; they are doing the delicate work of beading and making jewellery. You will read more about that in *Beyond The Storms*.

PART FIVE

God's Sustaining Grace
In The

STORMS

Grace Kept Me

I am alive today because God kept me. I am alive today because of His saving grace. He kept me. God kept me, so I would not give up. Grace secured me. Grace surrounded me. Grace sustained me. Grace held me up. Grace qualified me when I should have been written off and abandoned. I thank God for His amazing and unending grace.

> *Grace on the move.*
> *Grace in motion.*
> *Engraced.*

These were the new "names" given to me by my husband, my brothers, and a dear friend Sista. Overnight, my niece Gracie, had to share her name with me. The only response I could give to the many comments and questions about how I coped through the trials and travails of my soul over several years was that; I got to know God in a better way through the things I suffered—through my trials, challenges and difficult circumstances.

Abounding Grace

I got to know His rich and abounding grace. His grace strengthened me. Grace kept me through the thick and the thin. I

> **I got to know God in a better way through the things I suffered—through my trials, challenges and difficult circumstances.**

could have been dead and gone but grace kept me alive, and made me a living testimony. Grace kept me smiling and cheerful through pain and distress. Grace held my head up when the natural reaction would have been to stay bowed down in sorrow and disappointment. Grace did not let me go.

Amazing grace kept abounding to me. Praise be to God Who causes ALL grace to abound to us, that we having ALL sufficiency in ALL things, may abound unto every good work (2 Corinthians 9:8). Grace is God stooping down to reach out to us at our point of need. He is the God of all grace. After we have suffered for a little while, He will Himself restore us, making us strong, steadfast and firm (1Peter. 5:10). The grace of God within us enables us to labour more efficiently and abundantly for God. Grace fulfils a purpose in us and it enables us fulfil purpose and destiny. The ALL sufficient grace of God is available to everyone who is a Christian.

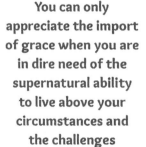

You can only appreciate the import of grace when you are in dire need of the supernatural ability to live above your circumstances and the challenges besetting you.

"The grace of God is the favour of God bestowed to man who does not deserve this favour" - Harold L. White.

As grace abounded in Christ and He went about doing good works, so also can the superabundant grace of God abound in our lives to do exploits for God and to bring about change in our situation, if we open our hearts to receive it even in our challenging circumstances. You can only appreciate the import of grace when you are in dire need of the supernatural ability to live above your circumstances and the challenges besetting you. Indeed, I can speak authoritatively on grace because I have an experiential knowledge of the sufficiency of the grace of God to sustain us through the valleys of the shadow of death.

"Grace abounds like an ever-flowing stream in the valley of adversity"

After one hundred and nineteen days in three hospitals, I certainly know more of God than I did before that one phone call on April 13th, 2013. I have a richer experience of God as a strong deliverer because of all I went through during this period. I know for sure that Jesus cares for me. I have been pruned and refined, and the process is still ongoing. My testimony is richer. I know what it means to be sustained by grace.

The Bible admonishes us in Hebrews 12:15 to see to it by looking after each other so that no one is to miss or fails to receive the grace of God. This grace of God changes lives. It sustains His children through the dark seasons of their lives. We have a responsibility to encourage one another to tap into that grace. This is the chief of purpose; to make evident the difference grace makes in our lives when we hold on to God to see us through every season of our lives—good or adverse.

"...Don't be conscious of (or focus on) what you are lacking (or in need of). Be conscious of (or focused on) God's superabundant grace for you and avail yourself of it" - JosephPrince.com (emphasis mine)

I am grace in motion.
I am grace on the move.
I am graced for good works and to do exploits for God.

I know that grace brought me this far and grace will lead me on. I am in awe of God for the grace that keeps abounding to me each day. Words fail me to express my gratitude to Him.

#

I Got To Know Him In A Better Way

Hardships, trials and challenges will come to us at one time or the other during our lifetime, if we are true sons of God. We must view them as God disciplining, correcting, pruning and refining us because of His love for us. We must be assured that His grace is available to see us through them all.

"Divine discipline is an evidence of divine love."

The Bible is replete with examples of many servants of God who endured hardships and we can see their outcomes as they were made strong to do exploits for God. Jesus endured the cross. Consider for a moment what He had to endure; the shame of the cross, separation from His Father, bitter hostility, grievous opposition from sinners and His visage marred beyond recognition (Isaiah 52:14). In considering what Jesus endured by going to the cross to die for our sins, we will not lose heart or grow weary as we run our own race and walk the path set before us.

God did not cause the disaster but He turned it around and worked it together to bless uncountable lives for generations after.

Hardships, trials and challenges will come to us at one time or the other during our lifetime, if we are true sons of God. We must view them as God disciplining, correcting, pruning and refining us because of His love for us.

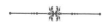

Some of Paul's letters to the churches were written while he was in the prison. He bore a thorn in his flesh. He did not have a wife. He was imprisoned, placed under house arrest, shipwrecked and finally martyred under Nero's reign. But he wrote thirteen Epistles that still give us divine direction today.

Many of the hymns and songs we love to sing today were composed following challenging circumstances in the lives of the composers. The first one that comes to mind is "It Is Well With My Soul" penned by Horatio Spafford after traumatic events in his life in 1871. The hymn which was inspired by the deep grief Horatio endured and at a time of intense sorrow is still touching lives and grieving hearts till today, more than a century later! God did not cause the disaster but He turned it around and worked it together to bless uncountable lives for generations after. I am particularly touched by the following lines:

> *Though Satan should buffet, though trials should come,*
> *Let this blest assurance control,*
> *That Christ has regarded my helpless estate,*
> *And hath shed His own blood for my soul.*

Whatever my lot, my challenges or difficult circumstances, God has taught me to say; "it is well, it is well, with my soul." This song ministered hope to me so many times during my storms. I knew through the experience of Horatio Spafford that none of our experiences is a waste. God is working out something through it that will bring blessings to lives somewhere down the road.

> **I can testify of the visions, dreams and ideas He birthed in me while I was buried like a seed in the ground beneath the surface. It was during my season beneath the surface that He caused my roots to grow deep down into His love.**

"Why should I be discouraged... When Jesus is my portion? My constant friend is He."

(A line from "His Eye Is On The Sparrows)

I got to know God better and deeper during my nights of pain and days of distress. I learnt to depend on His word as if my very next breath depended on God. I got to know the faithfulness of God in keeping His promises through all I suffered in the valley of the shadow of death. I got to know the amazing and indescribable love of God that He so richly poured out into my life when I knew that He was in the valley with me and He never for a moment left me alone.

We become more creative in our times of personal challenges and difficulties if we open our hearts to receive God's abounding grace available to us. I also can testify that through it all, I have got to know and experience God in a brand-new and intimately personal way. I can testify of the visions, dreams and ideas He birthed in me while I was buried like a seed in the ground beneath the surface. It was during my season beneath the surface that He caused my roots to grow deep down into His love.

#

Kept Again By The Power of Jesus

This chapter may well be titled "Kept by the Hands of God." But I have used that caption in an earlier chapter of this book. Indeed, it is the sum of my testimony. The phrase was inspired by the song sang by Mrs Toun Soetan during the 1990s while we lived in Ibadan, Nigeria. In fact, my husband and I almost played the life out of the cassette. He left it on every night so that it could continue to minister to our spirits, mine in particular, as I was going through both physical and spiritual assault from the devil in November of 1998.

I found myself humming the song several times during the night and day. It brought me untold assurance that I am kept by the power of Jesus. That was the original lyric: *"Kept by the power of Jesus, kept by the power of God. Day by day, come what may, we are kept by the power of God."*

This song inspired the signature statement in my email messages and on my blog; Enriching Lives. Inspiring Hope.

"Kept by the Hands of God, day by day, come what may!!!"

Naturally, it was the caption of the first blog post I did when I could write again after the restoration of my hands in July 2013. It was the only way I could summarize the events that had transpired in my life between April and June of that year, which I shared in the first part of this book. As I wrote the blog, my first son's middle name resounded in my spirit—Osemudiamen, which means "God is standing by my side." It was because God was indeed standing by my side and because He kept me by His mighty power that I was restored to the land of the living.

David in Psalm 30: 1-3 gave praise to the Lord Who delivered him from the place of much distress (from death).

"I will exalt you, O LORD, for you lifted me out of the depths and did not let my enemies gloat over me.

O LORD my God, I called to you for help and you healed me.

O LORD, you brought my soul up from the grave; you have kept me alive, that I should not go down to the pit."

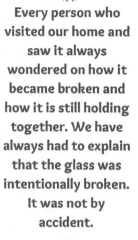

Every person who visited our home and saw it always wondered on how it became broken and how it is still holding together. We have always had to explain that the glass was intentionally broken. It was not by accident.

I could relate to these scriptures because it was the hand of God that lifted me out of the place of much distress. God heard me when I called on Him. He brought my soul up from the grave and He kept me alive.

#

Broken But Sandwiched in God's Hands

In 2004, my husband and I went shopping for furniture for our new home. We went with our very close friends, Bro. O and Sis B,

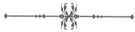

When I think of the many scars crisscrossing my body, I feel like my broken glass dining table. When I think of my new lungs, prosthetic limbs and many dental implants, I feel like I am made up of many broken parts put together by God with His own spare parts. But not only did He put me together, He is holding all the different parts glued together by His amazing grace.

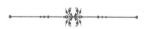

to serve as umpires. I was glad we did. I had colour scheme and aesthetics in mind. My husband was focused on functionality even if bordering on boring. We debated almost every selection before coming to an agreement. But there was one piece of furniture that we agreed on without any argument or debate. It was love at first sight for both of us. That is our dining table.

It is made of broken glass pieces glued together and sandwiched between two plain glass plates. This glass top sits on its stand without any screw but simply with its dead weight. It is a pure work of art. It bears its broken look but never falling apart. It has a greenish hue. This greenness symbolises for me a new beginning from a state of brokenness.

Every person who visited our home and saw it always wondered on how it became broken and how it is still holding together. We have always had to explain that the glass was intentionally broken. It was not by accident.

I have spent more time at this broken glass table than anyone else in my house. It is from the corner of this table that I have written most of the articles that I share to inspire hope. It is from my small corner on this table that I reach out to the world. It is my home-based office during the day and dining table in the evening and during the weekend. My broken glass table has been a source of inspiration to me in its brokenness—though broken it is standing very strong.

There is a new beginning arising from my season of brokenness.

When I think of the many scars crisscrossing my body, I feel like my broken glass dining table. When I think of my new lungs, prosthetic limbs and many dental implants, I feel like I am made up of many broken parts put together by God with His own spare parts. But not only did He put me together, He is holding all the different parts glued together by His amazing grace. I am sandwiched in His mighty hands. It gives me rest and comfort that none of the broken parts will ever fall away.

God's mighty hands keep me strong in my brokenness. I am broken but I am never falling apart. There is amazing strength exuding from my broken, tried and tested body. That strength has its source in my personal revelation and knowledge of God, Who works all things together for our good and Who is working in mysterious ways His wonders to perform in my life.

I am broken not by accident but intentionally by God's incomprehensible plans. His thoughts are not our thoughts nor are His ways our way. I have lost count of the number of times people ask me what happened to me when they see me with a walking stick. I am too young to need a walking stick, so something must be wrong. Upon my response that I am an amputee, they commiserate with me; "you had an accident?" They assume a woman of my age could only have become an amputee because of an accident. I have also lost count of how many times I have heard people ask, "what has lungs got to do with legs?" "How could a chronic respiratory disease result in the amputation of limbs?" Well, only God knows how amputation fitted into what He has planned for my life even before the foundation of the earth was laid.

There is a new beginning arising from my season of brokenness. A new thing is springing forth, behold it is now. With this broken vessel put together again by God and filled with His anointing, I am fulfilling purpose and working in the fullness of what God intended for me and created me for. The process of breaking me steered me into the path He had ordained for me. I did not envisage this event. Perhaps, if I did a few years back, I would have screamed my refusal to the highest heaven but what God is bringing out of the process is beyond my wildest imagination that I would not have wished for anything otherwise.

In my brokenness, I have learnt total dependence on God. A lesson I could never have learnt otherwise. I am still learning to rest my entire weight on God and on His unfailing love. My broken body is made whole because Christ's body was broken for me. It is the One who created me who defines that wholeness. In Him alone I have been made complete and perfect despite my brokenness.

As my green tone, broken glass top dining table continues to elicit amazement so also I know that my story and testimony of

God's amazing grace in my life will continue to elicit much praise to God and much wonder at His faithfulness. In which case, it would have been well worth the journey.

What more could I ask for when God has made me a wonder to many?

#

I fell Down But I Got Up
He got up so I could get up again
(SONG BY Travis Greene)

Nothing prepared me for the first fall. It was a freak and frightening accident. My stumps were still wrapped in the blue padded soft cast. It was barely two weeks after the amputation. I was sitting on a modified wheelchair that was extended to allow my stumps rest straight in front of me without hanging down. The extension was padded on both sides to safeguard my stumps.

The nurse had come to dress my tracheotomy wound, which had adhered to muscles around my trachea such that the hole was not closing as fast as it should. I had an open hole in my throat that needed to be dressed and covered. She had asked Sista Iy to leave the room, who was not particularly happy with the idea being a nurse herself and with the way the nurse had handled the wound previously. I pleaded with her to go for a walk. She did. And the nurse commenced. After a short while working on the wound, she realised she needed more materials, and had to exit the room to get what she needed. It took her a long while to come back. I was thirsty and needed a drink of water.

The cup of water was on the table that was usually beside me but the nurse had pushed it out of the way to allow her attend to me. It was out of my reach. So, I pushed my upper body forward a bit and stretched out to reach the cup. In the process, I shifted my weight on the extension attached to the wheelchair. The balance shifted like on a pivot, the extension swung downward with the load of my weight and in a split of a second I was on the floor.

An intense fiery pain shot through my right stump as I landed on it, the soft cast around the stumps did little to dampen the impact. The echo of the scream emanating from somewhere deep within my being reverberated from the room across the hall like the cry of a banshee. The nurses ran in one after the other with Sista Iy on their heels.

It was Michel who got in first, he must have taken in my body contoured in pain on the floor and in a flash, he was on his knees beside me. I was convinced I had fractured my amputated leg going by the waves of pain hitting me as if driven by gale force winds. Images of my amputated leg in plaster of Paris flashing in quick succession gripped my heart with fear intensifying the pain.

Michel and another nurse lifted me from the floor as all the other chorused, "*Qu'est que passé?*" In tears, I tried to explained how I reached out for the cup of water and lost my balance.

Sista Iy's face was as dark as a thundercloud. She looked like a Senior matron addressing a nurse caught making a colossal mistake in the management of her patient. "Why on earth was she left unattended?" The thunder clap echoed in the room. "This would never have happened if I had been here." She stumped out of the room while the nurses settled me in bed, gave me a quick check and called for the floor doctor. I wondered where Sista Iy had gone.

I asked her when she came back a short-while later. She had gone to look for the hospital administrator to report the incident. She was angry and hurt on my behalf at the same time. The walk around the hospital in search for the office of the administrator helped her to calm down and focus on supporting me to get better. So, she came back without reporting but still threatening to report the nurses. I was glad she had not report the incident to the hospital authorities. I had established a very good relationship with the nurses who cared for me for many years in that same ward and I did not want an administrative action taken against any of them.

After a series of checks and an X-ray, I was glad that there was no damage to what was left of my lower limbs. I was shaken by fear of a fracture and the impact of the fall. We managed the pain with medication and it improved subsequently.

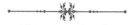

If I wanted to be independent and regain my autonomy, I knew I had to pick myself up, get up and keep moving forward. Staying in the place where I had fallen would definitely not get me to where I want to be.

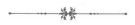

The next fall came while I was trying to dress up after my shower during my stay in the Rehabilitation Centre. It was on a Sunday. I was getting ready to go for my home visit. My husband and sons were coming for me after the church service. I wanted to pick a nice blouse for the home visit. Again, I reached out too far to the edge of the wheelchair to pick the blouse, the chair tipped over, and down on the floor I went. I laid crumbled on the floor with the wheelchair over me for a while, helpless and frustrated that it happened again

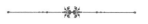

It is not over when you can still tap into God's strength. It is not over if you keep your gaze fixed on God and what He has planned for you instead of focusing on the place when you have fallen.

and on a day I was scheduled for a home visit, and I could not get myself back on the chair without help. I did not want the visit to be cancelled because of the fall.

I reached out and pulled red ball attached to a long white twine by the side of the wash basin next to the wardrobe to activate the emergency bell. The nurses were in the room in an instant. We played the scene again. "What happened?" They asked. I explained while they remove the wheelchair, lifted me back on the chair and wheeled me back to bed. The nurse wanted to be sure that I was not in pain. She wanted to call in the doctor. I assured her I was not in any pain. Only my nerves were frayed. She told me she would check back on me in one hour. She would let me go on my home visit if there was no pain or swelling. Thankfully, there were no swelling or visible bruises, and I was permitted to go home with my family when they came for me.

I continued the rehabilitation at home after I returned home fully on the 9th of August. I had two different physiotherapists coming to the house and the ergo-therapist still working on my hands. There was also someone who was supporting my re-integration back to home life and teaching me how to regain my autonomy at home. One of the things the physiotherapist taught me to do was how to get back up again if I fall at home and there is no one around to help me get up. It was a difficult process. It is still very hard for me to get on my knees when I have my prostheses on because of the difficulty in flexing my ankles.

The technique for getting up after falling required several moves; I have to drag myself towards a chair, move into a kneeling position in front of the chair, raise up one knee until the foot is flat on the ground and then push down on the raised knee, one hand on the chair and the other on the knee until I could slip my buttocks on the chair. This was the hardest part because all my weight must rest on one knee while pushing up with the second knee. I was glad I had learnt the technique by the time I had the third fall.

I was alone at home that day. It is not a strange thing for me to be alone. My husband was on duty travel. Ehi had gone to school. I had planned to go downstairs for breakfast after dressing up and putting on my prostheses, so I did not ask Ehi to leave a breakfast tray for me when he left for school. But that morning, my stumps were swollen. The volume did not go down after tying the bandage for over two hours. For a while before then, I was having increasing pain in the prosthesis because I was also putting back some of the over 30kg weight I had lost. I was hungry. I needed to take my medication. So, I decided to leave the bandage on and go downstairs to the kitchen on my knees. I had done that before many times but with someone at home to take down the wheelchair for me to move about with at that level until I was ready or could wear my prostheses.

> **"Are you going to leave behind a legacy that will continue to inspire lives after you are gone?"**

Since I was alone at home, I had to move one of the coffee stools to the kitchen so I could reach the cabinet with the breakfast stuff. I got the tea and the sugar out. I pushed the stool to the other side of the room while moving on my knees. I got back up on the stool again and knelt on it just as I did previously and reached out for the loaf of bread. I got it and set it on the worktop. My plan was to get down from the stool, move all the items on a tray, place the tray on the stool and push the stool to the sitting room. I missed the edge of the stool as I tried to get down, I slipped and landed on the kitchen floor. I sat there on the floor for a while, not quite sure what hurt me the most; the pain from the floor or the stark reality of life as an amputee. I once heard in a movie that every amputee knows that you will heal but you will never be the same again. That message was driven home as I laid on my granite kitchen floor.

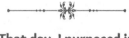

That day, I purposed in my heart to make God proud of me and happy that He gave me a second chance at life. I purposed to make my second chance at life count for something of eternal value.

If I wanted to be independent and regain my autonomy, I knew I had to pick myself up, get up and keep moving forward. Staying in the place where I had fallen would definitely not get me to where I want to be. What will get me to the place where dreams come true and purpose is fulfilled is to get back up again. Getting back up is the way forward and it does not mean I would not fall

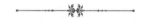

again. I have a few more times. Praise be to God who continues to keep my bones from being broken and whose grace abounds to get me back up again.

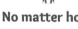

No matter how dire your situation may be, hold on to the faith, hold on to hope, don't give up on God. He will not give up on you.

It is not over when you can still tap into God's strength. It is not over if you keep your gaze fixed on God and what He has planned for you instead of focusing on the place when you have fallen.

#

A Second Chance At A Purposeful Life

That I had been given a second chance at life was not subject to debate in my mind. But that truth was driven home in a way that I could never have imagined and in a way that ensured that I will never forget it when I learnt of the home-call of my friend, Sally. I met Sally at the University of Ibadan, Nigeria in 1983. We later became part of the same circle of friends after I gave my life to Christ in 1984 and started attending the Ibadan Varsity Christian Union Fellowship.

Sally got married to Bro Bayo (as we called him then) in 1990 and they later moved to Chicago in the United States of America. They became Pastors of the RCCG Jesus House, Chicago. I was in a coma fighting for life when the Lord called Sally back home on Tuesday, April 17th, 2013. My husband did not tell me about it when I came back to the land of the living. I learnt later that he actually deleted every text message and email about the death of my dear friend from my cell phone so that I do not accidentally stumble on it until he deemed me ready to deal with the news. It was three months later when my brother, not knowing that my husband had not yet told me, informed me of his trip to Chicago. And I asked him what he went to do there. He knew Bro Bayo and Sally very well.

I was stunned by the news. I didn't even know Sally was ill. I was too caught up with all I was going through and was not following up well with my friends. That hurt me deeply; that she was so ill and I did not know about it. But much more than that I could not understand, how Sally who was ill for only six months could be called home at the same time while I who had struggled for many years with my health to the point of death was returned to life. I asked the Lord many times why He took Sally in and sent me back when we both stood at the pearly gate on April 17th, 2013. I pondered the more on this as I listened to Sally's last sermon on a YouTube video made by her church media to celebrate her life. It was in September 2012, just before she was diagnosed to have colon cancer. It was moving and illuminating. The sermon was a preparation for her home-going.

She said, "It is appointed for man once to die, then after that judgment."

"There will be a rising from the dead. There will be a resurrection of the dead."

"I hope you are assured that there is life after death."

Sally imparted lives in many ways. She was a wife and mother, an educator, a mentor and an encourager to name a few. She believed strongly in the institution of marriage and counselled many. My Maid of Honour, Muyiwa, who was very close to her, told me that she was at peace at the end of her life. She had the assurance of eternal life in Jesus Christ, who she served faithfully since she got born again at the age of 14 years. She left behind a legacy of love and zeal for God.

"Are you going to leave behind a legacy that will continue to inspire lives after you are gone?" Her message echoed at me for many days after I watched the video. Would I leave a legacy of eternal value behind when the Lord calls me back home? I knew at that instant that God has given me a second chance at life so that I can live purposefully and impact lives of people in every sphere of my influence.

Sally's death affirmed to me that I was given a second change to live purposefully. There is life after death. There is coming a glorious day when we will exchange this physical body that is subject to disease, pain and affliction for a glorious incorruptible body. Therefore, we need to make assurance doubly sure that we hold on to the faith and hope we profess until the end, and that we are ready to meet our Lord and Saviour Jesus Christ when He comes for His own.

There is nothing more important to me in life than to hear, "Well done, my faithful servant" when I appear before the throne of glory at the end of my sojourn here on earth. That day, I purposed in my heart to make God proud of me and happy that He gave me a second chance at life. I purposed to make my second chance at life count for something of eternal value. I determined that I would relentlessly pursue and accomplish the purpose for which God has spared my life; I will deliver glory and honour to God. So, I prayed again that God will make me an inexhaustible conduit of His blessing to as many as He will bring my way, and recommitted my life to Him to do with as it pleases Him and in accordance to His call upon my life. It is imperative that I fulfil and accomplish what God has called me to do here on this side of eternity. That is what will give God pleasure and bring glory to His name.

> After a few days back at home, I was quick to realize that our definition of normal had changed. We had to implement several changes in the way we do things in order to accommodate the changes that had taken place in my life.

If God gives me the chance to look back after He eventually calls me home, I want to see on the day people gather together to celebrate my life; many people who would testify that their lives were touched for good because I lived. I want to see people dressed in white and with a touch of orange and green, not mourning but rejoicing that I lived my second chance at life purposefully. I desire to look back and see amputees who walked because I lost my feet, widows who had because God made

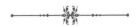

"you can choose to be angry with God for what you have lost and what you cannot have again or you can choose to be thankful for what you had, what you now have and what you can still have if you entrust your life into God's hands

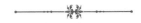

me a Dorcas for them, and people who did not relinquish their grip on hope because God used the narrative He creatively crafted of my life to inspire hope in them and encourage them not to give up.

No matter how dire your situation may be, hold on to the faith, hold on to hope, don't give up on God. He will not give up on you. Ultimately, heaven is the reward of those who hold on to the faith to the end. Don't miss it. There is nothing worth missing heaven for.

#

A New Definition Of Normal

It was with exhilarating joy that I walked into my house on Friday 9th August, 2013, after one hundred and nineteen days stay in three hospitals. I was back home to stay and not on a day visit. Many things had changed; the three oxygen reservoirs were gone. And there were no more blue tubes lining the stairway and the floor in the sitting room. The ventilator was gone. Hallelujah! It was pure joy. This was a landmark moment, an evidence of God's ability to grant us the desires of our hearts and answer our prayers. I wanted to be back

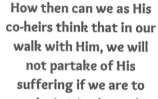

How then can we as His co-heirs think that in our walk with Him, we will not partake of His suffering if we are to partake in His glory when it is revealed? We also being sons of God are not exempted from suffering, challenges and changes.

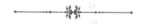

home before my son, Ose, returned to school in the United States. He had left me in the hospital the previous year, he came back to meet me in the hospital and spent his entire summer vacation by my bedside. Each time I asked him to go and spend time with his friends; his response was that it was his choice to stay with me. I did not want him to leave me in the hospital this time around. I desired it. We took it to the Lord in prayer. And the Lord granted me the grace and strength to accomplish all the targets and milestones my doctors and physical therapist lined up for me. They could not find a single reason not to let me go back home after a three week stay in the Rehabilitation Centre. It had never been done before that a bilateral amputee would spend just three weeks in rehabilitation. God again made me a wonder to many. He made me an evidence of the working of His amazing grace in the life of His children.

The following Sunday, with joy exuding from our grateful hearts and from the hearts of our friends, we were received back into the church. I walked to the altar and with my family beside me, we gave thanks to God for keeping me alive and for bringing me back into His house. We sang "Praise My Soul The King Of Heaven," a hymn that has become the Family Anthem of the Williams Family. We sang "I Am A Living Testimony" by the Mighty Clouds Of Joy, a song I heard on my way for my home-visit the previous week and it resonated with me. I could sing again. God is truly wonderful.

> Through this new definition of normal, we are equipped to fulfil our God-given purpose and destiny.

I noticed another change, we were not in a hurry to leave church immediately after the service, because I was running out of oxygen. We could wait after the service, and spend time to sharing fellowship with the brethren and our friends. All praise be to God.

Dealing With Change

After a few days back at home, I was quick to realize that our definition of normal had changed. We had to implement several changes in the way we do things in order to accommodate the changes that had taken place in my life. There were moments in those early few days that I felt overwhelmed by these changes. At such moments, I had to quickly remind myself that I have been singing, "I could have been dead and gone, but You kept me living on. I thank You, Lord, I'm still alive."

Change comes to us in diverse way through our experiences and, sometimes, through the challenges we face. It could be the death of a loved one, ill-health, loss of a job, loss of limbs, broken relationships, change in location, failed project and accidents to name but a few. In most cases, we are not given time to prepare for change. It could take just a phone-call.

Things may never be the same again after such change. I watched the movie "Courageous" shortly after I got back home from the hospital. In it, the Pastor said, while counselling the grief-stricken Mitchell whose nine-year-old daughter just died, that "dealing with grief is like dealing with an amputation. Because every amputee knows that that you will heal but you will never be the same again." This hit me like a thunderbolt because I know just how true that statement is. I will heal physically and emotionally, in fact at that time, I was making good progress on the path of healing, but I will never be the same again. There will always be an empty space beyond my stumps whenever I take off the "feet of grace."

"My life has been a non-stop roller coaster ride of faith-building and character-refining trials." God's sovereign hand and control over my life has often placed me in humbling circumstances.

As I adapted to the new phase on my life, I knew that there are some things that will never be the same again. A major change had occurred in my life. As the Pastor, I mentioned earlier also said, "you can choose to be angry with God for what you have lost and what you cannot have again or you can choose to be thankful for what you had, what you now have and what you can still have if you entrust your life into God's hands." I can never have my natural feet back, certainly not the ones I had before, but I choose to be grateful for the life I have now and what God is working out though my experiences.

Ultimately, your change, whatever it is, can become a change for good depending on your attitude and your posture towards God, because God always works all things together for our good. Job had to deal with a massive change in his life, after the loss of his children, property and health, but nowhere in the entire book was it recorded that he was angry with God that he charged God foolishly. Notice his posture of resignation to the sovereign will of God in his period of adversity (Job 1: 21-22).

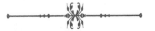

At such times when the storm of adversity is fierce and intense, it can be too much to bear. Even the most righteous will find it hard to hold back some grumbling and murmuring. It takes grace, divine strength and the knowledge of God's love for you not to focus on the challenges and the little irritations that seem to mushroom the more you think about them.

Learning To Persevere

In recent times, it is becoming obvious that often Christians are ill-prepared to endure hardship or to persevere through challenges. As soon as something goes wrong and not in accordance to their expectations, they get angry with God and become sour in their attitude. Jesus learnt obedience through the things He suffered, and He is the Son of God. This experience made Him to be perfectly equipped to become the Author and Source of eternal salvation (Hebrew 5: 8-9). Christ's sonship did not exempt Him from obedience, suffering or change.

How then can we as His co-heirs think that in our walk with Him, we will not partake of His suffering if we are to partake in His glory when it is revealed? We also being sons of God are not exempted from suffering, challenges and changes. These are instructive in deepening our knowledge of God and by them we learn experience. If we endure with Him, we will also reign with Him (2Timothy. 2:12). We cannot learn perseverance if we have no reason to persevere. We cannot learn to be steadfast during trials if we are not tested. Neither can we learn patient endurance if there are no challenges to endure. The seasons of adversity that we go through give us the opportunity to develop our spiritual muscles so that we can add patience, perseverance and endurance as virtues to our faith.

The Bible encourages us to add all these qualities to our faith so that we can become fully matured. It is only when we possess these qualities in increasing measures that they will keep us from being idle and unfruitful in our knowledge of Jesus Christ. Whosoever lacks these qualities is short-sighted and spiritually blind. We are therefore admonished to be all the more eager to make our calling as Christians sure. Perseverance, patient endurance and steadfastness are essential qualities for fruitful Christianity. They only come through what we suffer when we go through trials and testing. All these bring about changes in our lives. They define a new normal for us.

He is a God given to details. Not one single event in our lives is purposeless. It is like a piece of a jigsaw puzzle, which has a definite place to occupy for the final picture to be complete.

Through this new definition of normal, we are equipped to fulfil our God-given purpose and destiny. This song by the Brooklyn Tabernacle ministered to me in one of those moments when I felt overwhelmed.

> *For every mountain You've brought me over.*
> *For every trial You've seen me through.*
> *For every blessing, hallelujah;*
> *for this I give You praise.*

Whatever change is taking place in our lives, let us tap into the superabundant grace of God as you learn to persevere through it by applying Biblical truths and standing on the authority of God's irrefutable promises.

#

For A Purpose And A Reason

There was an overwhelming response from family and friends when I could write and blog again and I shared snippets of what had transpired in my life during the almost three months that I was "hidden away" underground. Many of the responses had one message in common beyond joining me to rejoice and give thanks to God, and that was, God has a grand plan for my life.

I have pondered on this truth repeatedly since I was restored to the land of the living. The more I pondered on this, the more I knew I must take time to dwell in the presence of God to seek His face to make His grand purpose plain and clear to me. I knew I needed to have clear instructions and directions

I have learnt that being the Beloved of God does not grant us immunity from sufferings, tests and trials

from God as to where He is leading me in this second chance at life He has given me.

In agreement with Rosann Cunningham of Christiansupermom.com, I can say with definite conviction that; "My life has been a non-stop roller coaster ride of faith-building and character-refining trials." God's sovereign hand and control over my life has often placed me in humbling circumstances.

The many years of struggling for breath; the fear of not knowing when things could suddenly go wrong; the numberless long stays in the hospital for over twenty years; many times, flat on my back and confined within four walls; then the season of oscillating between the bed and wheel chair; the loss of independence and autonomy and being at the mercy of others were just a tip of the ice-berg of the storms of adversity I weathered for over twenty years. On top of these, watching our finances wiped away and being unable to earn an income was one of the most difficult challenges for me to bear. I cried many times watching my husband bear up under the burden and helpless to support him in a tangible way. Then unexpectedly, I became an amputee. That was more than the last straw, which but for the amazing grace of God would have broken the camel's back.

At such times when the storm of adversity is fierce and intense, it can be too much to bear. Even the most righteous will find it hard to hold back some grumbling and murmuring. It takes grace, divine strength and the knowledge of God's love for you not to focus on the challenges and the little irritations that seem to mushroom the more you think about them.

Not surprising, once you get into that mode of grumbling, complaining and indulging in self-pity, the enemy will bring more stuff to irritate and distress you. So, what do you do? I tell you, I have had a sizable share of this inward struggle. It takes grace, grace and more grace not to go off track like a derailed train with devastating effects, such as despair, despondency and discouragement.

Things can get to the point where you cry out, "I have had enough, I can't take any more." It did for me many more times than I can count. Even Prophet Elijah went through such a valley of discouragement and despondency. But see the way God ministered and revealed Himself to Elijah at the lowest point in his life. He also revealed the purpose He wanted him to fulfil (1Kings 19).

At first, when I contemplated on the limitations the loss of my limbs imposed on me, I was confused. I was angry. I wanted to know why. I felt I did not need that additional complication in my life after all I had been through.

Amid the emotional struggle dealing with the amputation, like I mentioned earlier my Sistafriend, Bidemi, said to me, "No one expects you to be a super Christian, you can approach God and tell Him how you feel, you can ask why, and you can pour out your heart before Him. He is your Father, He will wrap His arms around you and comfort you." That was exactly what I did. He did wrap His arms around me, and He speak His peace into my heart, giving me the assurance that what He is about is beyond my wildest imagination.

It is at such times that an understanding of God as a God of purpose becomes a life-saver. The storms I have weathered are for a purpose. I was processed and refined to fulfil destiny. I once wrote a blogpost titled; *"There is purpose in the process."* That message came alive to me in that period after the amputation, I had to read it again and again. I determined in my heart not to miss the comfort God has for me through this situation. Most importantly, I was reminded that it was not about me, it is for the glory of God to be put on display in my life and for many lives to be impacted and touched for good.

My husband and many others encouraged me; "Focus on the victory God has given you and all He brought you through. Keep the ultimate goal in view, that is fulfilling your God-given purpose," they said to me. I had come too far to give up in that season. God gave me the special gift of grace to regain my cheerfulness and to remain positive and focused. Having such an assurance that God's dealings with me are for a reason and a purpose was a great encouragement.

He ministered to my heart that the amputation would only be a limitation if I allow it to be. He told me He has given me the feet of grace to break away from the restrictions and to enable me fulfil His calling upon my life. We have a choice to view God by our situation or to view our situation through God.

God of Purpose

There is a divine purpose for everything that happens to us in life. I know for sure that there is a reason for the experiences and rough roads God has taken me through. Because I know God is a God of precision. He is a God given to details. Not one single event in our lives is purposeless. It is like a piece of a jigsaw puzzle, which has a definite place to occupy for the final picture to be complete.

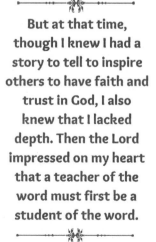

Stormie Omatian wrote on her Facebook page; "Don't let the storms of trials, struggle, grief, or suffering (affliction), make it hard for you to see what is ahead. There is always a place of calm, light, clarity and peace to be found, if you will take God's Hands and let Him lift you above your circumstances into His rest, comfort and protection."

But at that time, though I knew I had a story to tell to inspire others to have faith and trust in God, I also knew that I lacked depth. Then the Lord impressed on my heart that a teacher of the word must first be a student of the word.

Amid our trials and sufferings, we can be assured that it is God's purpose and counsel for us that will prevail (Proverbs 19:21). God's plans stand forever and the purpose of His heart remains through all generations (Psalm. 33:11, NIV). Job said, "God performs His plans for me." What He wants to do is what He does (Job 23: 13-14). God is unchangeable (Hebrews 6:17). He is working out His purpose in us when He takes us through the rough path.

"God's purpose for me is definite, unique and unchangeable."

Because of the inability of God's purpose and plans to change, we who are called to inherit the promise can have indwelling strength and strong encouragement to hold fast to hope appointed for us (Hebrews 6: 18). This hope is an answer for our soul, holding firm and secure through our trials and struggles.

"Hope is the light shining in the darkness of disappointment." - *Sarah Young (Author, Jesus Today Devotionals)*

Jesus walked the rough path to the rugged cross at Calvary to reconcile us to the Father. On that rough path, He was beaten, spat on and jeered at, yet He did not utter a word. He is our perfect example.

I have learnt that being the Beloved of God does not grant us immunity from sufferings, tests and trials. If we are heirs of God and co-heirs with Christ Jesus, we must of necessity suffer with Him, if we are to share in His glory (Roman 8:17). I have also learnt a deeper depth of hope and faith through my tests and sufferings.

"Faith is a mindset that expects God will act no matter what happens, no matter what I may be going through."

I know that I am going to the nations, that much has been impressed upon my heart. The more I dwell in God's presence in obedience, the more He will reveal His plans for me. He will give me step-by-step directions. I wait with great expectation for God's grand design for my life to unfold.

My stumps and prosthetic limbs keep me in constant touch with my limitations, and constantly reminded of my need to depend on Him to do what only Him can do through me.

Whatever you may be going through at this moment, don't give up, hold fast to hope, God is working out His purpose in you. Be assured that God has a unique and unchangeable plan for your life, if you will trust Him with your life.

\#

Remodelled
(He is the Potter and I am the Clay)

Earlier, I explained that I love sitting at the dining table with broken pieces because it reminds me so much of me held in my Father's arms. The table was made just like the clay pot. That clay pot was sun-baked when the Potter made it. The pot had some cracks in it but it still held water and served the purpose of the Potter for a time. One day the Potter picked up the clay pot and said, "I know the plans I have for you. My thoughts for you are higher than where you are right now." Then He showed the clay pot a vision of what He had in mind for it. The clay pot was excited, "I like what you have in mind for me, Potter. Do with me as it pleases you." The pot had no idea what dangerous prayer it had prayed.

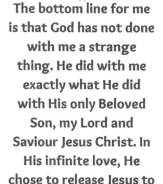

The bottom line for me is that God has not done with me a strange thing. He did with me exactly what He did with His only Beloved Son, my Lord and Saviour Jesus Christ. In His infinite love, He chose to release Jesus to be the first to be broken, and He was broken for you and me.

"I will, I surely will." The Potter responded and He smashed the pot on the rock. The broken clay pot cried out in agony. "What are you doing?" At the command of the Potter, the whirlwind of affliction blew upon the smithereens, it whirled and swirled them like a centrifuge would. The Potter picked up the smithereens left behind after the whirlwind of affliction had passed. He melted them and remoulded it into a vase and fired it in the furnace of adversity. "O Potter, this is too much. How much more can I take?" The clay pot wailed and cried out in agonising pain.

But the Potter responded, "My eyes are intent on you. I am with you and will never leave you alone." He did not take His eyes off the pot in the fiery furnace, no, not even for a split of a millisecond. He kept His gaze focused on His pot. At the right time, He brought it out of the furnace, and just before cooling, he broke a piece off the rim of the vase. He broke the piece off at a point that will always be in the line of vision of the vase. It cannot be missed. He painted and decorated the porcelain vase, filled it up and set it ready for use.

And the vase asked, "Oh Potter, why hath thou left me thus?"

"You are mine," said the Potter. "I have chosen you for a task that you cannot complete on your own. I broke off this piece to keep you reminded always that you are Mine. So, that you will always depend on me to fill you up and pour you out as it pleases me. My grace will always be sufficient to keep and sustain you."

The porcelain pot was certainly more beautiful than the clay pot. It has a different purpose to serve for the Potter than the clay pot. The clay pot had to go through the process required by the Potter to become the porcelain vase the Potter desired for it to become.

The wonderful works of God puts His glory on display in our lives.

I was that clay pot. It was either late in 2002 or early 2003 that the Lord confirmed His calling for my life. He impressed on my heart that He has called me to be an Inspirational Speaker and a teacher of His word. I was very excited about the vision He gave me and I desired to operate in that calling. God opened an opportunity for me to minister at the church I was attending then in Tamale; the Lighthouse Church International. My Pastor and friends asked me to minister during one of the Sunday Services. I spent time in God's presence to receive a message from Him for His people and I prepared as best as I could to bring His message to His people. But what transpired on that day was beyond my imagination. I felt like I was out of my body watching from the side-lines. God's power moved in our midst to touch the people in a way I could never have imagined. I was tingling for days afterward. I must confess that one part of me was very excited about what I saw God do through me and wanted more of it. But at that time, though I knew I had a story to tell to inspire others to have faith and trust in God, I also knew that I lacked depth. Then the Lord impressed on my heart that a teacher of the word must first be a student of the word. I knew that I was not the kind of student of the word that He wanted me to be yet.

It was from that moment that He took the clay pot, me, and broke it. He passed me through the whirlwind of afflictions, to the extent that I reeled and was giddy at the force of the wind. But He did not stop there. He put me in the furnace of adversity. That was where I learnt that God will never use a vessel He had not thoroughly tested and refined. The process of refining was intensely painful. But I had the assurance of His presence. I knew His eyes were intent on me. I knew that He is such a good Father who would never let His child cry without a reason. This assurance many times took the sting out of the pain. No matter how long the night may be, I knew the Lord will come through for me and the dawn will break. The promise of a new day will bring with it new possibilities and new experiences of God's sustaining grace through the storm.

When I was told that my legs were to be amputated, I found it very hard at the beginning to comprehend how this could possibly contribute to the glory of God being displayed in my life. After everything I had been through—the whirlwind of afflictions and furnace of adversity, I had to ask - what more does the Lord want to do with me by taking away my legs. I found solace in the word that He gave to us through our friend that He will give me the feet of grace that will take me to places beyond my imagination, places my natural feet could not have taken me.

He remade me into the kind of vessel that would be fitted for His Kingdom agenda for my life and He did it in such a way that I could never be puffed off because I am always reminded that I belong to Him and He does with me as it pleases Him. My stumps and prosthetic limbs keep me in constant touch with my limitations, and constantly reminded of my need to depend on Him to do what only Him can do through me.

I know first-hand how Paul must have felt about the thorn in his flesh, especially, when he understood of the purpose of the thorn. It was to keep him from becoming conceited, proud and puffed up because of the great power of God being manifested through him and the greatness of the revelations God gave him. It kept him from being excessively exalted. It kept him humbled and glorying only in his weakness so that the strength and power of Christ may rest on him.

God knows me well enough to know that I would need a constant reminder of His grace to keep me in check, to keep me from becoming too elated at the things

But there can be no testimony without a test. And it does not matter how long the tests and trials last for.

He would do through me, and to know that everything He does through me is simply for His glory. And He would not share His glory with any man, least of all me. I guess, I can also say that I know myself well enough to know that I needed such a gigantic billboard announcing that it is the hand of God that kept me this far and it is His grace that is sustaining me. I am certainly reminded every morning when I swing my legs out the bed each morning and I get on my wheelchair to go to the bathroom. I am reminded of God's sustaining grace each time I put on my "feet of grace." I am reminded each time I am supported to climb on to a podium that grace is what is keeping me afloat as I minister God's message of hope to His people. It is this understanding of

God's purpose for my handicap that keeps me grateful for it. Because I now know that many things that the Lord is doing through me could not have happened in this dimension if He had not taken that piece off the porcelain vase. Now, I no longer see on my preparation process as a handicap but I appreciate it as an essential gift that has made me better suited for God's purpose.

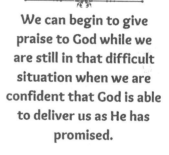

We can begin to give praise to God while we are still in that difficult situation when we are confident that God is able to deliver us as He has promised.

He remade me into a porcelain vase that will always look up to Him for leading and depend on Him for guidance to perform the assignment and the good work He called me to do even before the foundation of the world was laid.

The process of going from clay pot to porcelain vase was not easy but it was needed to prepare me to fulfil God's purpose and calling on my life. It is a process I would not exchange for another. The bottom line for me is that God has not done with me a strange thing. He did with me exactly what He did with His only Beloved Son, my Lord and Saviour Jesus Christ. In His infinite love, He chose to release Jesus to be the first to be broken, and He was broken for you and me. It was God's good plan to crush Him and make His life an offering for sin, so that God's good plan will prosper in Jesus hands. If God can allow Jesus to be broken, He certainly can break me too. This is the reason why I can trust God and it is the reason why I can trust Jesus. He experienced it all before He called me to have a taste of it. I can trust God to break me because He is the One Who made me. And He knows how to remodel and remake me. Each one of us must be broken at one point in time in our life or the other, so that we can become fully yielded and fitted for God's use.

So I am fully persuaded in any situation we face in life, no matter how long it has lasted; God is working it out to put His glory on display in your life.

God holds the pieces of all that has been broken in His mighty hand and not a single piece is lost. But they are all fitted together to display the awesomeness of His power. They are wonderfully put together to display His glory. And at the end of it all, God only is honoured and glorified.

I pray that my life and your life will bring glory and honour to God in every way, in Jesus name.

When God Puts His Glory On Display

Do you remember the old Sunday School chorus based on the healing of the lame man by Peter and John at the temple's gate called Beautiful in Acts 3?

Silver and Gold have I not
But such that I have give I unto you
In the name of Jesus Christ of Nazareth
Rise up and walk

He was walking and leaping and praising God x2
In the name of Jesus Christ of Nazareth
Rise up and walk.

The crippled man rose up, he walked, and leaped and praised God. The people around the temple saw him walking, leaping and praising God. And they recognized that it was the same man who used to sit at the temple's gate begging for alms. They were filled with wonder and amazement at what had happened to him. Note that, the man was crippled from birth.

The wonderful works of God puts His glory on display in our lives. People and nations, including the heathen, shall see it and declare that our God is good. When God moves on our behalf at the appointed time to show pity on us and to favour us, people around us shall see it and worshipfully revere the name of the Lord. Kings shall praise Him because of His mighty works in our lives (Psalm 102:13-15).

Great was David's distress and affliction in Psalm 102 that he sat alone like a bereaved sparrow on a rooftop. He was inwardly depressed by his afflictions and trials that he lost the will to live.

But David was confident that God will answer his prayers because he knew that God will not despise the plea of the destitute. He was confident that God would not forget, forsake or abandon him.

For the Lord looks down from His Holy heaven to behold us His people on earth, and to listen to our plea. Because of His faithfulness to us, men will declare His praise and people shall gather together to worship Him. It gives me such an assurance to know experientially that God looks down from heaven and He beholds us. His eyes are intent on us and He is greatly concerned about us. David was assured that because of the anticipated deliverance, the name of the Lord will be praised when the people of God gather together in Zion.

This same confidence and assurance was expressed in Psalm 126 as he declared: "When the Lord turned again the captivity of Zion, we were like them that dream." God did an amazing thing in our lives to the extent that it was like a dream. It was too good to be true. Because of this awesome work of God, we are laughing with joy and overflowing with praise. Our praise is loud and copious that even the heathen (that is, those who don't believe in God) around us, who hear us have to affirm that our God had done great things for us.

It is simply delightful when the display of God's might and faithfulness in our lives would cause even those who do not acknowledge God to declare and confirm that our God is good and worthy to be praised. When God gives us a testimony that requires explanation, everyone who sees us will acknowledge the faithfulness of God on our behalf and give praise to His Holy name. That was the case for me on the first Sunday of December

2013. It was the Annual Thanksgiving and International Day in church, a day we set apart to bring offering of thanks and praise to God in a truly multicultural and international way. We are from different nations and cultures, and we add this diversity to our celebration of God's goodness in our lives. It is usually an extended service followed by a food fellowship during which we share food from our different countries to wrap-up the celebration.

It was an exceptional day of exhilarating joy for me for many reasons. Remember, God has done great things for us, whereof we are glad. First, it was the first Church Thanksgiving Service that we did not have to worry about having to send someone back home to refill the oxygen tank because we would not have sufficient oxygen for the whole period we had to be in church; the journey takes about 45 minutes to go and come back. In 2012 during the same event, my husband who is the choir leader had to leave mid-service to dash back home and refill the oxygen bottle.

Secondly, there were people at this special service who had not seen me for over a year. The joy they expressed when they saw me without the supplemental oxygen paraphernalia was indescribable. They were so glad for me that they kept praising God and thanking Him for my healing. I was truly overwhelmed at their reaction. They had never seen me before without the paraphernalia. It was a unique sight for them. One of them was the Guest Preacher. He surely gave praise to God for what He has done in my life and he declared that this is a testimony that needed no explanation.

But there can be no testimony without a test. And it does not matter how long the tests and trials last for. It is the victory that God gives us over the difficult and challenging situations that brings the praise and puts the glory of God on display in our lives. Like the man who was blind from birth and was healed by Jesus in John 9, it was for the glory of God to be made manifest that he had to go through that difficult situation. Our calamities and afflictions are for the glory of God and to make manifest His works.

In Matthew 9:8 and 15:31, the people were amazed, astonished, awestruck and they marvelled when they say the dumb speaking, the maimed become whole, the lame walking and the blind seeing. These are testimonies of the power of Jesus to heal at work in the lives of these individuals which could not be hidden. Then the people praised and glorified God. That power to heal and to deliver is still at work today in the lives of those who put their trust and hope in God, and believe in His name. It worked in my life and made me a living testimony of God's faithfulness.

What we need to do in our day of trouble, distress and affliction, is to call upon the name of the Lord. As He promised in Psalm 50: 15 and 23; He will answer us and He will deliver us. And what should our response be to this? We praise and glorify His name. But that is not all, many people around us will see it and give praise to God because of what He has done for us. David anticipated God's deliverance. He was very confident that God will not leave him in his difficult situation; therefore, he could declare in advance that God will be glorified and praised because of what He will do on behalf of His people. We can begin to give praise to God while we are still in that difficult situation when we are confident that God is able to deliver us as He has promised.

We can praise our way through our days of trouble and distress just like Paul and Silas praised their way out of the prison. See the number of lives touched because these men confidently praised and worshipped God even while in bondage and shackles. God was so moved that He had to step into their situation and that cause the earth to quake bringing about their deliverance and release.

So I am fully persuaded in any situation we face in life, no matter how long it has lasted; God is working it out to put His glory on display in your life. It is possible, you feel as if God has abandoned you or He seems too far off, and you have not seen your desires fulfilled yet. Be assured, this situation is for the glory of God to be revealed in your life. One thing I am confident of is that God loves you passionately with an amazing and unending love, and He is daily putting that love on display in your life.

Look back, look around you and then look up. There is so much for which you can thank and praise God now. And soon, at the fullest of time, God will put His glory on display in your life such that men will see it, they will marvel, and they will rejoice and glorify God because of you. This assurance alone is a reason and an opportunity to rejoice in the Lord and be glad. His word is that those who sow in tears will come again with rejoicing and exhilarating joy as they bring the sheaves in.

When the power of God is manifested in our lives, the people around us will be gripped with great wonder and awe. They will praise God on our behalf. And they will proclaim that they have seen an amazing and extraordinary thing—things you would not normally expect.

That is what God does with the story He writes of our lives; He uses it to cause us to acknowledge His glorious works in our lives.

PART SIX

Leaving Footprints despite the STORMS

Our Lives as Testaments

———— ▬ ————

This section would have been left out or included somewhere else under comments and reviews from family and friends. However, I needed to include it in my journey of faith because even though I had hinted at it in the book, it was important for me to stress once more that our lives matter to God. Not just because He wants to receive the Glory due Him but because after all is said and done, our lives are the testament to the fact that He is real. We often expect that the testaments of faith ended with the Bible but it continues today with the written and unwritten stories of our lives.

Our lives are a proof of this God that we have chosen to serve through the valleys and the mountains, the darkness and light – a proof of His unending love for us and humanity. They serve as a roadmap for others to follow, others to find God and in other cases to encourage others. The stories of faith in the Bible were written to do all of these things and more and indeed, our lives continue the story from where the Bible ends.

Throughout the years of storms, while I was visibly concerned about what each event was doing to my family especially my sons on an emotional bent, I never quite gave thought to what they saw every time they looked at me. It never occurred to me, that in my own way, I was living the Faith I had professed to them ever since they were young children.

But the thoughts that have poured out of these wonderful God-fearing young men have left me in awe of God and the handsome gifts He has committed into our care and also provoked me to ask – As you live through each calm, each storm and sometimes windy climes and other times cyclones, what picture does your life paint to your family, your children and friends? A picture that you indeed "Love and Serve a living God" and are irrevocably loved by Him or a picture that your declarations of faith do not go beyond your lips? These are a few of mine. Are you leaving any footprints behind?

A Message From My Son, Ose

3 years ago today Mom, you came home after spending 119 days in the hospital!

In those 119 days;

You had a lung transplant that caused your body to completely shut down forcing you to be in a coma for a month.

Your feet and hands died, but your hands came back to life and you learnt how to write all over again.

You went through an amputation of both your feet and had to learn how to walk with Prosthetics.

But through all that you set a goal of coming home before I left for school and you surprised all your doctors and achieved that goal.

In the three years that you been back home from the hospital, you have achieved so much more than I could have ever imagined.

- You completely mastered walking and living with prosthetics to the point where you have walked in two 5k walk events.
- You have started a beading business, making beautiful jewelry with the hands that came back to life.
- You have started an amazing non-profit to raise money for amputees in poor regions of the world who would have never gotten the chance to own prosthetics/wheelchairs.
- You are traveling the world and attending conferences where you motivate and inspire people with your story.
- You have created an active inspirational blog that is being read by people all over the world.
- You have prepared a book for publishing and have been featured on a TV show.

And I'm sure that there are many more things that I'm missing!

I'm sooo proud of you mom! You proved all the time that anything is possible with God and the right mindset!

Thank you Dad and Ehi because without everyone's support this family would not have achieved nearly as much as we have!

Message my Son Ehi wrote on my last blog post before I went into the hospital, on the day coma had to be induced. The second message, a post on his Facebook wall...

Message 1:

He was with you yesterday. He is with you today and FOREVER will He be.

We love you, Mum

Message 2:
Not many of you know, but my mum used to have a chronic respiratory disease called bronchiectasis and a debilitating neuromuscular disease called myasthenia gravis. Both diseases weakened her lungs. She coughed terribly every day for 20 years unable to breathe well. At a stage it came down to her needing to get a double lung transplant. As a result of the complications following the surgery, she ended up having both her legs amputated. She now walks with prostheses, but has been traveling all over the world sharing her story and promoting the charity foundation she started.

The Feet of Grace Foundation raises funds for people in developing parts of the world (currently just Nigeria) who are unable to afford the high cost of prosthetic limbs and have, therefore, lost access to a lot of things in life.

This is the second year that we are having the Hit the Street for their Street event, a 5k walk-athon, and I like to do a mini version out here in Claremont. My plan is to do a 2.5 mile walk around the 5C, taking about an hour.

PART SEVEN

Connecting The Dots With Appreciation

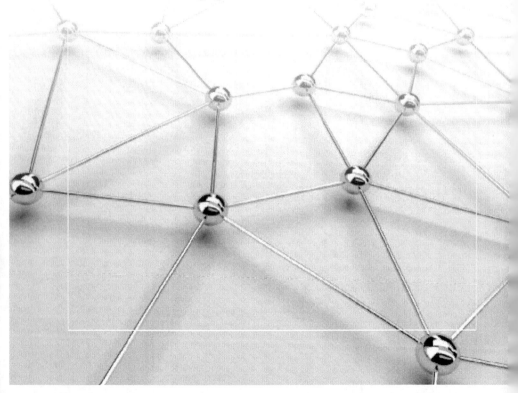

Connecting The Dots With Appreciation

The Beginning of My Story

My life story is like a page in a connect-the-dots puzzle book except that mine has many unnumbered dots. My feeble attempts to connect the dots failed woefully because the One who laid out the dots is infinite in His creativity, wisdom and knowledge. His thoughts are beyond my thoughts. Be that as it may, there are significant connections made as God gave me the revelation, which left me in absolute awe of His awesome greatness. Being persuaded that God is not haphazard in His dealing but very meticulous with great attention to minute details, I pay attention to every dot and connections in the landscape of my life.

I made my entrance into the world on Saturday, October 1st 1966 at the Jericho Nursing Home, Ibadan, Oyo State, Nigeria. My mother's labour was long. I was overdue but it was God's plan for me to arrive on October 1st. It is not a coincidence but by God's crafty design that my 50th birthday and Jubilee celebration fell on a Saturday. Jericho Nursing Home became a significant landmark in the landscape of my life as time went on and as you will find out. Needless to say, I know that I am a Nigerian by God's purposeful design, being born on the sixth anniversary of Nigeria's Independence Day.

I was born to Rt. Revd I.B. Williams and Mrs O.M. Williams. My father named me, Irene Titilola Oluwatosin. Irene means peace in Greek. I later found out that Irenic means promoting peace, conciliatory and facilitating reconciliation. I have seen these attributes play out in many instances in my life.

My father was a minister of the Methodist Church of Nigeria from where he retired as a Bishop. My mother was a School Teacher. With a preacher for a father and a teacher for mother, I had a very strict upbringing. Going to church was what we do every Sunday. It was not an option. My most vivid childhood experience of church was at the Olowogbowo Methodist Church in Lagos. My love for hymns was ignited by the Choir of that church. Many times, during my seasons of adversity, I recalled several the hymns and special songs by the Church's Choir, which are indelibly etched in my memory. We lived in the Church Manse on Bankole Street. The one-story house with potted rose garden on its veranda holds many memories for me, some good and some not so good, which inspired my first fictional work in progress. I started reading my father's collection of the Royal National Rose Society's magazines at the age of 8 years old, and fell in love with roses—alive or dead.

My father promised me a legacy that no man can contest in any court of law. He gave me a legacy of sound education up to the post graduate level. He drove me to and from school until I was 12 years old. My mother taught me the power of a praying woman long before a book was ever written on the subject. I remember the bedtime stories she read to us. One of them remained vivid in my memory. It was the story of the little girl who lost her penny, and her mother asked her to pray about it. She did, and she found the penny after praying. That has remained a constant reminder each time I lose something; I take it to God in prayers. My mother taught me the value of hard work. She constantly reminded me that hard work does not kill. She exemplified resilience in the face of adversity. I am eternally grateful to my parents for the foundation they laid for who I have become today and for the roles they have continued to play in my life. These experiences of our lives as a family have shaped me in many ways beyond what can be described in this book.

My Primary school education was at Ereko Methodist School at Beckley Street in Lagos. My earliest recollection of my life's story started from the dual-level apartment we lived in, on top of the headmaster's office when I started primary school. The screened balcony overlooked the sandy quadrangle where the assembly was held every morning. It was just a walk down the stairs by the side of the building and I was in school. My mother taught in the same school but I was never placed in her class. Memories of the School headmaster, Mr. Banjo, the sandy quadrangle, brown khaki uniform and the almond fruit tree in front of the school inspired my first published story, *I Crossed The Street*, in the Anthology of the Geneva Writers Group – *OffShoots 12 Reflections*.

There were four of us at that time; my brothers Ibukun and Olaleye, and my baby sister, Mary Olujoke. It was the year she was born that I stopped playing with dolls. I had a red feeding bottle warmer to turn on and a baby to feed. By that time, we had moved from the apartment above the school to a bungalow behind a very big house at Apapa Road, Ebute-Meta, Lagos. My mother brought my baby sister to school with her in the afternoon. I went back home with her after school while my mother was teaching in the afternoon session. It was my responsibility to care for her until my mother got back home.

I was baptised at the Methodist Church, Ebute Meta. After the Baptismal Service and still in my white frilly frock, I rode my bicycle along the gravel path in front of our home off Apapa Road, behind the Agip Petrol station and the Military hospital. That picture continues to amaze me because I cannot imagine myself astride a bicycle now. I will never forget the day my little brother, Olaleye, went missing from the house and was found more than 500 meters further down the Apapa Road. God has been watching over our family for a very long time. This was before we moved to the Manse at Bankole Street, Olowogbowo on Lagos Island. Each house we lived in during my childhood is a significant thread woven into the tapestry of my life, each of them with its unique stories.

My childhood was not protected from the winds of adversity as I watched my family packed out of the Church Manse in the heat of the Methodist Church conflict in 1976. I heard the stories through the thin walls. I heard the whispers of pain, anguish, anger, frustrations and disappointment that transcended beyond the church conflict to places a child would have considered safe. We moved from a mansion to a two-bedroom bungalow in Itire, and I knew all was not right. Not with the early morning guests to our home who brought with them more pain and anguish. Soon after, Ibukun and I went to live with the Mr and Mrs Sonekan, and their son Lande in Ikoyi. They were my parents' friends from church. We went to school from there and went back home every Friday for the weekend. I remembered the dinners of banana fritters and plate load of fried plantain, dodo. I called them my foster parents. I am grateful to God for the role they played in my life during that season.

Tolulope, my third brother and number Five, came in March that year. And I saw first-hand how wicked a fellow human being could be to another as my brother went through harrowing experiences in the hands of the nanny who had the duty to care for him. Oluwaseun, my forth brother and number Six, came in November 1979 and we moved from the small bungalow where I entered puberty to a yet-to-be completed mansion at Obanikoro. The house was my training ground for adulthood. I learnt advance courses in child care and home management in the five-bedroom house. By the time I exited that house, hard work and multitasking became second nature to me. I formed lasting relationships in that neighbourhood, especially with Bolanle Zubair. Together, we oscillated between our houses at both ends of Jolaoso Street like a yoyo during school holidays to the chagrin of my mother and her step-mother. We walked back home from Secondary School together almost every day.

My secondary school education was at the Methodist Girls' High School, Yaba, Lagos, from 1977 to 1982. Mrs Moji Oni (my mother's senior at the Teachers' Training College) took care of me in her home after school while I waited for my father to pick me up. Mrs Onafowokan and Mrs Pearse along with many other teachers instilled discipline, diligence and pursuit of excellence in me. I am greatly indebted to these women for the deposit they made in my life at that formative age. *In Love Serve One Another* was the motto that has continued to compel many of us old girls of MGHS to forge a relationship that lasted over more than three decades since we left school. *Must Gain High Standard* became our motivation. It was at MGHS I met my birthday twin,

Adeyinka Ogunnaike, who has become a champion for my cause. I am truly blessed to call her, "My Twinnie."

I did a stint of A' levels at the Federal Government College, Odogbolu, Ogun State in 1982, while waiting for admission into the University of Ibadan. It was short and sweet, a bridge between protected life at home and the unrestrained liberties of University life. But I had the opportunity to put my French into good use there. An old family friend was there with me, Olukemi Oluyede nee Kuforiji. Her parents were my parents' close friends. She protected me from the "seniors."

I cannot recount my childhood stories without noting our relationship with the Akinyemis and the Sondes. These were the two families apart from the Kuforijis; we were sure to visit during weekends and holidays. Their children were the only friends we had growing up. Their parties were the only ones we attended. Mrs Akinyemi was my mother's friend from Teachers' Training College. They taught together at Ereko Methodist School until she went home to be with the Lord in 1979. Mr Doye Akinyemi is akin to an uncle to me and to my siblings. His first daughter, Akindotun Merino, is my first and longest friend. She has remained my sister by another mother. Her brother, Soji lived with my family in Obanikoro during the 1980s after the death of their mother. The twins, Kennie Okh and Taiwo Benson, and their brothers, Tunde and Folabi are all in my tribe. Though separated by distance for many years, we have managed to forge a deep relationship. These connections have taken a vibrant dimension to touch many other lives as we sought to be Agents of Change for our generation.

University of Ibadan was an experience extraordinaire, where significant events took place to shape the course of my life. I met Prof. Abiodun Johnson, a Professor of Paediatrics and my father's very good friend. He and his wife, Aunt Regina, provided a home away from home for me in the university. I got my first pair of high-heeled shoes from Aunt Regina. Uncle AOK was instrumental in directing me towards Human Nutrition as a course of study when I did not make the requirements to study Medicine. He remained an Uncle figure for me. I can never thank him enough for the extra miles he went on my behalf and for the many times he allowed himself to be used by God to pave a way for me. His second daughter, Damilola, is part of my tribe of "cousins."

I spent the first two years in the university with an attitude of carefree and unrestrained freedom. It was free at last to do what pleased me after the restricted upbringing I had. This carefree careless life left scars that will remain with me for life. During these two years, I forged a lasting friendship with Yomi Aliu, Aderonke Denloye and Ebun Arimah. I did a 180 degree turn around in August 1984 when I made the decision to accept the Lord Jesus as my Saviour. I had attended the Vacation Youth Fellowship at the Oritamefa Baptist Church, Obanikoro, at the insistence of my brother, Ibukun. He had become born again earlier, and was relentless in his pursuit of me. The message preached that night grabbed hold of my heart. "You must be committed" rang in my ears all the way home and would not let me go to sleep until I fell on my knees by my bedside in the middle of the night. I asked God to forgive my sins and I turned over my life to God, accepting Jesus Christ as my Lord and Saviour.

I began a personal relationship with God. He was no longer just the God of my father and mother to me, He became my God. I joined the Ibadan Varsity Christian Fellowship and pursued my love for music singing with the Jesus Revolution Voices. That was where I connected with Sis Toyin Aransiola, who is now with the Lord. She took me under her wings. I met Victor and Tolu Okoruwa, Emmanuel Salako, Abraham Ayelabowo, and Matthew Ayoola among others, who all helped me as I grew in the Lord. I desperately needed new friends to cheer me on in my walk with the Lord. My old friends were holding me back to the life I no longer wanted to be identified with. That was how Tola Dawodu, Funmi (Sally) Adewole (now home with the Lord), Mowunmi Osinubi, Shade (Shandy) Ajayi, Toyin Morakinyo, Yinka (Smiler) Adelaja, Bola, Ronke Ajav and many others got woven into the tapestry of my life. These ladies helped to me to draw closer to the Lord. Thank you all for remaining great friends to date.

It was during a Christian Musical Concert with the Calvary Love Singers (UCH Christian Fellowship) at the Paul Hendricks Hall, University College Hospital, that I crossed path with Peter Olumese in December 1984. I saw him on the stage with his lanky body bent over his bass guitar, which he still plays with passion till today. We became friends and that was all there was to it for the next five years.

In 1985, my fifth and last brother, Olakunle, made his entrance into the world. After recovering from the initial shock, I shifted to the opposite end of super excitement. I had his photograph on my table in my hostel and in my wallet. I took him everywhere I went when home on vacation. This earned me some explanations some years down the road.

I finished my first degree in Nutrition in 1986 but not before making another significant connection. She was my senior colleague in the Department of Human Nutrition. We were in the same research team under the supervision of Prof. Tola Atinmo, who as time went on became more of an uncle than a supervisor to me. I will always be grateful to Prof. Tola Atinmo for the role he played in my life especially later in my academic and professional pursuits. Dr. Iyabode Adeyefa took me under her academic wings and mentored me. She eventually became my big sister from another mother. It is amazing how God wove her into the tapestry of my life. Sis Iyabo proved herself to be a worthy big sister through the years. She midwifed many significant connections for me. She is truly the best I could have asked for as a Big Sister and friend.

I did my National Youth Service in Niger State. Orientation camp was at Bida Polytechnic. A stickler for time, my father got me to the orientation camp two days before it was scheduled to begin. He drove from Lagos all the way to Bida. As we passed Kainji, we remembered our family vacation at the same location earlier in the Seventies to visit the Carters. Then, my father drove his sky-blue Volkswagen Kombi van. I remembered our Christmas with the Carters' many cats. It was the first time I saw gaily wrapped Christmas presents under the Christmas tree like in the story books I had read. There was a gift for everyone in the family including the workers, and even the cats. Cats getting Christmas gifts was a wonder to me. But that vacation ignited my desire to bless others with gifts. Now I keep a gift box for all occasions. The Carters would never know the significant impact they made on me.

We arrived too early for the Orientation and there was no accommodation arranged for early arrivals. Because my father had to return to Lagos, he was compelled to seek alternative accommodation for me. Not wanting to leave a 20-year-old young lady alone in the hotel, he began to search for a Methodist Church. We found none. Next on the list was a Baptist Church. We found one. He sought out the Pastor of the church. He explained our dilemma and requested on the strength of his being a fellow clergy that they consider accommodating me for the night. They agreed and offered me a room in their very humble abode. My father ensured I was installed in a safe place before he departed for Lagos. That left a huge impression on me. The couple offered me dinner of guinea-corn meal and dried okra soup after my father left. I had never eaten such a meal before. Both the meal and the soup were dark brown. I could not refuse it. My mother taught me to always eat what is set before you. I ate it out of respect and honour to them. This Baptist couple taught be an invaluable lesson by their willingness to put a roof over a stranger's head simply because they considered us as one in Christ. In doing so they helped to shape another significant piece of the puzzle that will eventual fit at its rightful place in God's plan for my life.

I left Niger State to continue my Youth Service in Lagos when the strong winds of affliction blew wildly over me in November 1986. It was a close call and narrow escape. But in the process, the attending House Officer at the Lagos University Teaching Hospital while taking history of past medical events, inadvertently gave us an insight to the pattern of the storms. I knew at that instant I was not wrestling against flesh and blood but against powers and principalities, and spiritual wickedness in high places. God used Koye to open my eyes to what was going on. We remained friends for a while before losing touch as we pursued different life goals. But that connection remained a significant part of my story.

In November 1987, I returned to the University of Ibadan to commence my Masters' degree in Nutrition. But it was not only a postgraduate degree I pursued, I had to review several spheres of my life. One of them was not heading in the direction I thought was God's will for me to pursue. I was hanging in a limbo and needed to take a decisive action. It was painful but necessary. By the time, I got my Masters in Human Nutrition in November 1988, I needed the time to heal and to be ready for what God intended for me. My stay in Alexander Brown Hall in UCH afforded me the opportunity to forge deeper relationships with friends who have remained important part of my life including Muyiwa Idowu who became my Maid of Honour and Moji Ajayi, who along with her husband, Sam, are friends my husband and I can count on. They are truly dependable friends.

Continuing straight on to do my PhD seemed to be the logical next step after my Masters. This quest brought me in close contact with experts with vast experience in both Clinical and field Research, including Prof Babatunde Oshotimehin who co-supervised and provided support for my doctorate research. Sis Iyabo midwifed many of these connections. Her office at the Metabolic Research Unit in UCH became my base and it was in that laboratory that I conducted most of my research work. I grew my fledgling research management and coordination wings during that season. It was also a place of many visitations from my friend, Peter, who was then a Resident Doctor in the hospital, and who often offered to give me a ride home.

My academic pursuits took me to the Dunns Clinical Nutrition Unit, University of Cambridge in 1989, where I conducted the literature search for my doctorate research work. But beyond, academic pursuits, I experienced the generosity of my friend, Ayodele Adenekan (nee Elemide), who housed me during my stay in London while I worked to earn the money I needed to support myself while in Cambridge. I worked in a New York Deli shop near Soho off Oxford Street, serving pastrami and rye sandwiches. I worked in a hospital as a maid cleaning and clearing patients' dishes. I worked in a restaurant washing dishes. Those were the days I thanked God for my parents who taught me that there's dignity in labour. An old missionary couple provided me with a bed and breakfast accommodation at a reasonable price in Cambridge. It was an attic room. Breakfast was toasts and tea. I soon found out that this sweet couple had once worked in Nigeria, in Ilesha, Osun State. I will always remember their kindness to me. Nnenna Frank-Peterside who was my neighbor in Queens Hall in the University of Ibadan during my final year in the University remained a dear friend to me during my sojourn in UK. Ayo's apartment at Saltram Cresent in Queens Park, SW London was the meeting point for old friends from university days, a place of many laughter and memorable events, including my brief romance with jerry curls. Church was at Kensington Temple, many of the melodious praise and worship songs I learnt there remained etched in my memory resurfacing in times of great adversity.

I returned home in December 1989 to continue my research work while at the same time working on a project facilitated by my academic mentor and supervisor, Prof Tola Atinmo and Sista Iyabo. It was on arrival back home after my six-month sojourn in UK, I noticed that something had changed in the dynamics of my relationship with Peter. It was no longer platonic and the usual light banter. It was becoming intense. My emotions were kindled. The opportunity of the National Nutrition Survey not only provided me with a timely escape from Ibadan but also was my first contact with UNICEF, the organisation sponsoring the survey.

I needed the space and time to seek God's face about the stirring in my heart. I was not willing to invest in another relationship if it was going nowhere, not after investing almost four years in a previous relationship. But God had a definite plan and a hand in this one, which would unfold beyond my wildest imagination in the years afterwards. On a Sunday afternoon, the sun was set to begin its drop and the sky was blue with scattered balls of cotton, Peter asked me if I would be his wife and the mother of his children. I answered yes. That turned out to be the best decision of my life after I gave my life to Christ. The day was April 29th, 1990.

My tribe began to expand after that day as I met Peter's parents; Mr and Mrs S.I. Olumese who I fondly call Papa and Mama. These ones are heaven's special gift to me. They are God's answer to the prayer I learnt to pray since I was 16 years old when I learnt the power of prayer from my mother. They have loved me as one of their own from the day I met them. Then I met Peter's sisters now; Anthonia Ameh and Pauline Osamor; and his brothers, Mark and Sylvester.

In the continued of pursuit of academic excellence, I left to the Department of Clinical Nutrition, University of Toronto to continue the laboratory work required for my doctorate research.

This connection was midwifed by Dr. Yomi Akanji. It was also an opportunity to develop an enriching relationship with Ebun Arimah, my good friend from the days in Idia Hall. We spent many Saturdays and Sundays together to kill the loneliness of being away for our beloved so far away in Nigeria in the days when there were no cell phones or emails, and letters take two to three weeks to arrive at destination. We scoured shops together as she supported me in the preparation for my wedding.

My tribe expanded even the more as my brothers and sister got married. It now includes Shalewa Williams, Foluso Williams, Oluwole Eni-Olajide, Funmilayo Williams, Blessing Williams. It expanded even the more as my sisters and brothers in law got married and Moses Ameh, Dr. Jon Osamor, Florence Olumese and Olanike Olumese were added to my life. My tribe includes my nieces and nephews; Jeffery, Chidima, Fiyinfoluwa, Babalola, Inioluwa, Bukayo, Holly, Gracie, David, Darasimi, Abimbola, Feranmi, Eseose, Perfect, Daniel, Oseremen, Esther, Ayomiposi, Idiahi, Sabaoth and the many more I am waiting for with hope and great expectations. My tribe extends to my cousins with whom I have maintained a thriving relationship; you all know yourselves. Every single member of my tribe has played a significant role in my life that will remain etched in my memory. I am blessed to have you in my life.

There are many more that God has brought into my sphere of influence especially my daughters in the Lord. Some are my friends' daughters, some have lived with me for a season, some were a timely help when most needed and some have been placed in my life for a unique purpose; Iranlowo, Faith, Olaoluwa, Ibukunoluwa, Mimido, Nguveren, Remi, Banke, Irene N, OluwaLaanumi, Leah, Valerie, Celine, Semilore, Gbemisola,

Dukia, Oluwafikayomi, Kristen and Marissa. They have given me a taste of what it means to have daughters while I wait for my Ruths to come. It has been an honour and a joy to be a small part of shaping these ladies' lives. Emmanuel was added to the mix in 2015.

Faith, Seyi, Titilopemi and Chioma were charged to remind me of my unfinished writing assignment. They had my permission to constantly ask how much I accomplished each week towards birthing the dream of writing my story into a book. The thought of giving an account to those who hold me in high esteem gave me the impetus to keep writing even at most challenging times.

Forging Connections:

It is an impossible task for me to note all the connections God has given me the grace to forge in the fifty years of my existence. Some have left such an indelible mark that I must not fail to mention them.

I am grateful for the Pastors, Fellowship Leaders and the Ministers who facilitated my spiritual growth at Shepherd's Hill Baptist Church, Lagos; IVCU, Ibadan (Pa Elton, Prof. Adesogan, Emiko Amosuka, Moses Aransiola, Dr. Durojaiye, Friday Bekee and many more); Chapel of Resurrection, UI (Revd. Ibeagha), Oritamefa Baptist Church, Ibadan (Revd. Leigh); Full Gospel Businessmen Fellowship; UCH Christian Fellowship; Christian Corpers Fellowship (Bida, 1986); Christ Chapel, UCH Ibadan (Revd Sam Omokhodion and the Pastoral Team); Lighthouse Church International, Tamale Ghana (Pastors Patrick and Joy Bruce); RCCG Victory Center, Geneva

(Pastors Carl and Patricia Shipley); Maadi Community Church, Cairo; and Tower of Refuge Church International Geneva (Pastor Edwin Idemudia and Dr. Funke Bolujoko). There are many men and women of God who have enriched my life over the thirty years since I came to know the Lord through their ministries via the Television and Internet for whom I give thanks to God.

Dr. Akin Eni-Olorunda and his wife who I fondly call, Sis T, were our prayer partners for many years after we got married. We spent many Sunday evenings praying for our families either in their home or at ours. Their first son Otito will remain ever fresh in my memory. IfeJesu, their last son is in my tribe.

UNICEF connected me with many people with whom I forged a long-lasting relationship. One of them is Adesoji Tayo and his wife Lara. What began as a professional relationship, working together to fight for the welfare staff grew into a relationship knitting the two families. Soji and Lara have provided a place for us to rest and recuperate in their home in Ibadan since 2008. It has been a home with all the needed support. They have been a tremendous blessing to my family that words fail me to describe our debt of gratitude to this wonderful couple. They, their children and siblings are part of my tribe. Even more significant is that every time I turn into the road leading to their home next door to Jericho Nursing Home, I am reminded of the place where I made my entrance into this world. How amazing God is to provide a place of rest for us next door to where I was born.

Adesina Adegunle has been a connector and financial adviser since we were in UNICEF. My husband and I have forged a thriving relationship with him and his wife, Toyin, who provided a platform for the Feet of Grace to reach people I could never have imagine reaching under one roof. Dr. Iyabo Olusanmi, Mrs Justina Onifade, Godwin Nwabunka, Olushola Ismail, Sola Adeyomoye and many more are some of the lasting relationships I forged through the UNICEF Nigeria connection.

Promoting Exclusive Breastfeeding brought me in contact with Babafunke and Fisayo Fagbemi, and their organization, Staywell. We joined forces to spread the message of the benefits of breasting and with our personal testimonies. That connection has grown into a deep and lasting relationship extending beyond our generation to our children.

When I needed a second opinion about my doctors' diagnosis in 1998, I knew I have friends I could call upon to help me out. They did not even tell me about their own storms until I landed in Columbus, Ohio. The first stop after they picked me up from the airport was the Neonatal Intensive Care Unit to see their pre-term twins. I didn't even know they were expecting twins. Wale and Kemi Sobande proved themselves to be true friends and burden-bearers when the doctors at the Ohio Medical Centre confirmed the diagnosis and gave me their report. They helped me through a difficult season while going through a difficult period in their own lives. I give praise to God each time I see their twins today.

It was Joy Bruce who came to my hotel room to welcome me to Tamale and invite me to their main church after she learnt that I had attended one of their parishes earlier that Sunday. That was truly a warm welcome. Our spirits clicked and that began a lasting relationship. Our boys soon became friends, and their home became our second home in a strange land. Pastors Patrick and Joy Bruce stood with me through the stormy whirlwinds of affliction in Tamale and took care of my children when I could not. Through this lovely couple, I made friends with many young men and ladies that have remained in my tribe to date. Pastors Patrick and Joy were the first to tell me that I have a story to tell and I need to write it in a book.

I made significant connections in Ghana, which are still thriving until today. Ernestina Agyepong was colleague Nutrition Officer and she became a friend who has remained a part of our lives. She has been a tremendous blessing to me. Karen and Maame have are significant connections in Ghana that I will never forget.

Coming to Geneva gave my husband and I the opportunity to make a significant connection and forge a relationship with Dr. Olumide Ogundahunsi and his wife, Sis Bola. I had met Sis Bola earlier while in the Department of Human Nutrition at the University of Ibadan and she went to MGHS for her A' Levels but I did not connect with her there. We had our Doctorate Graduation on the same day. The men shared an apartment at Serviette and Liotard streets. The wives and children visited on holidays. As often as we can, Sis B and I make quick visits to check on our husbands' welfare. We have many stories of lives shared together in brotherly love and most significant of these, is the support they have been to us and how they stood with us through the stormy seasons. Their home was home to our sons when my husband and I were away from home and when I had to be in the hospital. They stood in the place of big brother and sister for me on countless occasions.

Our relocation to Geneva and fellowship at the RCCG Victory Centre brought me in contact with Bro. Godson and Sis

Catherine Etitinwo, Sis Caroline Ezebunwo-Okere, Bro. Offei and Sis Dina Dei, Bro Atsen and Sis Liz Ahua, Bro. Godwin and Sis Gloria Enwere, and many others with whom we have forged a thriving relationship. These ones were there for us when we needed friends to wade the rough seasons with us. They are friends who stood in the gap and prayed with us and for us. My family owe a debt of gratitude to Bro. Godson who facilitated our settling down in Switzerland and has been an ever-ready help in navigating the administrative maze of the country.

It was at the Victory Center that I met Sis. Cynthia Samuel-Olonwonyo. She told me one day in 2004 after she heard a bit of my story that I need to write a book. She simply echoed the words of Pastors Patrick and Joyce Bruce. I knew at that time that I had the three witnesses I needed for the word to be established. She is a sister after my heart.

Mrs. Phebean Owolabi, Mrs Omo Eyo and Mrs Janette Awanem left an indelible mark on the tapestry of my life. These three ladies whose husbands worked with the Nigerian Mission in Geneva, came to my home and managed my kitchen every week for more than a year. They cooked many delicacies for my family at a time when the toil of the affliction compelled me to relinquish my strong hold on my kitchen. Many of the ladies earlier mentioned supported me by taking care of my husband and children when I could not. I will never be able to thank them for their kindness to me and to my family.

My sojourn to Egypt brought Vijay and Florence into my life. Vijay was my Section Chief at the UNICEF Cairo Office. We became and have remained great friends. They supported me through the difficult season in Cairo. Femi and Tayo Kupoluyi are one of a kind. I met them at the Maadi Community Church. At the time the storms roared against me in Cairo, this couple took me into their home, someone they knew for only months, and they took care of me until I left Cairo in January 2008. I am forever grateful to them.

We came from different Nations with different skin colours but we were bound together by the love of God and by our firm belief that there is power in the prayer of mothers. Together, every week we joined our faith and hands in prayers as we pray for our husbands, our children and their school. It has been a blessing to have Francie Namigai, Amy Wulf and Lisa Underwood woven into the tapestry of my life. We not only prayed together, they were there for me when I needed support and help to get to my appointments and get important things done. In the same group were Kim Zint and Rachel Garry before they left Geneva. We have continued to stay in touch and to pray for one another and our children.

My path crossed with Dr. Adebisi Adebayo in Geneva. In the bid to find an alternative source of income after separating from UNICEF on health ground, I connected through her with Maryam Moghalu and Ekene Guy-Okafor, who is now home with the Lord. We marketed Mary Kay Cosmetics together and developed a relationship that transcended marketing cosmetics. A relationship that we have maintained through the tough seasons we have both weathered.

My first contact with Effectual Magazine in October, 2010 was divinely orchestrated when a dear brother in church blessed me with an enveloped gift after the Sunday service. I opened the envelop and found in it a copy of Effectual, a Magazine for women and those who love them. It was of high quality both in content and presentation. The colours were vibrant and inviting. The message was richly inspiring. I was deeply impressed, specially noting that it was published in my dear country, Nigeria. It took another two years and seven months of building a relationship via phone and by email, and waiting with expectation before I finally met in person Bidemi Mark-Mordi, the Author of Sistapower and Publisher of Effectual Magazine. So much transpired in between. She had been in my home with her husband while I was in coma. My connection with Bidemi and her husband, Pastor Mark Mordi has led to a thriving relationship between the two families, which has been a tremendous blessing to us. Through this relationship my tribe has extended to include Coach Anna McCoy who challenged me to finish my book, Audrey Joe-Ezigbo and the Sistas across nations. These Sistas inspire me to be strive to be the best God has created me to be.

We came to Tower of Refuge International Church in 2011 and forged a deeper relationship with Pastor Edwin Idemudia and his family, Dr. Teju and Dr. (Mrs) Funke Bolujoko, and with Deboh and Bhola Akin-Akintunde beyond our initial connections. I am grateful for the support and encouragement the Pastors, Leaders and members of the church have provided to my family. The Bolujokos became the Uncle and Aunty we can count on to be there for us. They have been a tremendous blessing to our family in many more ways than I can recount. Aunt Funke and I can spend hours on the phone talking. She is a woman whose quiet resilience and dedication inspires me. The Akintundes are friends indeed. Bhola's dedication and sense of duty is admirable. I am grateful to God for the multifaceted and deepening relationship I have forged with her.

Many thanks to Laurent and Evelyn Zbinden, and Lorraine and Gamis Missatou for the role you are playing in making the **'Beyond The Storm'** part of our story a reality that is touching lives for good. Lorraine, your commitment to praying for us on every trip touches our heart.

My husband and I connected with Dr. Wilson and Robinah Were through the men's work relationship. Our relationship has grown deeper with each member of the family championing my cause. I am grateful to Robinah for the constant reminder that I need to finish this book and to Marissa for appointing herself as the Feet of Grace Foundation in her school.

From the foregoing, it is obvious that I can write another book to acknowledge all the persons God has brought into my sphere of influence who have made an impact on me. In fact, so many have touched my lives for good in many diverse and varied way. It is not an act of omission not to have mentioned each of them individually. I simply have run out of pages to do so. So I dedicate the words of gratitude below to every single man, woman, and child who has impacted my life and left an indelible mark of goodness on me.

Grateful For My Tribe:

Here I am Lord, ministering gratitude for the blessings of Family and Friends who makes up my tribe
I am grateful to You, O Lord, for blessing me with my Family and Friends
Family and Friends who have made me pause several times in a day to shout praises to You.

Thank You Lord for my Father and my Mother
Thank You Lord for Papa and Mama
Thank You Lord for my siblings, and their spouses, my nieces and nephews
Thank You Lord for my sisters and brothers-in-law and their spouses
Thank You Lord for my nieces and nephews
Thank You Lord for my cousins near and far.
Thank You for my longest friend of over 40 years.
Thank You for my most recent friend.
Thank You for friends I have not seen for up to 20 + years but have remained true.
Thank You for friends I see and talk to regularly but have learnt not to take for granted.
Thank You for friends I am yet to meet physically but are truly a blessing.

I am so grateful, Lord for Friends who have sown seeds of goodness into my life.
Friends whose acts of kindness have left indelible marks on me.
Thank You for friends who stood strong me when the going was rough.
Friends who wiped my tears.
Friends who comforted me.
Friends who knew when to be silent.
Friends who encouraged me.
Friends who would not let me give up.
Friends who did not let me go.
Thank You for Friends who laugh with me and who make me laugh out loud each day.

Thank You for friends who gave sacrificially time, energy and untold resources, and are still doing so.

Friends who have been a conduit of Your blessings to us.
Friends who opened their doors to me and to my family, some at short notice, some consistently for many years, some when we were in a strange place and they didn't even know us before, and some I am yet to meet but have been a blessing to my family.

Thank You, God, for many Friends who looked after my husband and sons when I could not. They cooked. They cleaned. They did school run. They did grocery. They ran endless errands.

I bless You, dear God, for Friends who prayed with great fervency when the clarion call was raised. They held fast to the horn of the altar. They gave themselves no rest until this daughter of Zion was delivered. Many didn't even know me personally, yet the prayed because Friends asked them to do so.

Thank You for Friends who have been destiny helpers, who champion my cause and speak out for me.
Thank You for Friends cheering me on in my race.
Thank You for Friends who have gone home before me.

Lord, I thank You for my dearest, truest and best friend, with whom I learn daily what it means to be truly one in You. Peter, you are the best I could ever have asked for as my husband. I am forever grateful for your love.

I thank You, Father for blessing my life with Peter Osemudiamen Oluwadamilola and David Ehimenmen Oluwatosin. My sons are a special gift from Your throne of grace to me. Thank You so much, Lord for these fine young men I am so proud to call my sons.

Thank You for my Unknown Benefactor who have me the gift with which you have kept me alive to this day.

Above all, I thank You for the Greatest Friend ever known Who loved me so much that He gave His life for me. The Lover of my soul. My Sweet Jesus.

Thank You Father God for blessing me with great Friends.
One thing I ask for today is that You bless my Friends with the good measures, pressed down, shaken together and running over. Please give them the grace to run their race to the end.

Thank You, Lord.

PART EIGHT

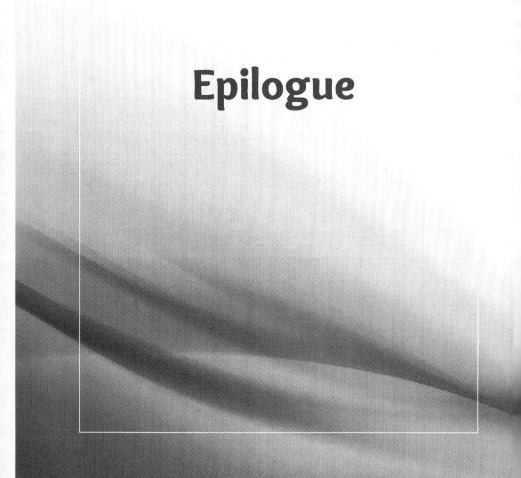

Epilogue

Epilogue

A Carefully Scripted Narrative

If I could write the script for my life myself, I would certainly have edited out the twenty long years of rib-cracking and painful cough. I would have deleted the years of distress highlighted with the burden and shame of affliction. I would have penned a much shorter and less tortuous route to my healing. I would have inserted an instant and spectacular miracle of healing at the laying on of hands by a renowned Servant of God. There would have been no chapter on amputation and life as an amputee.

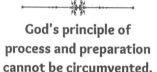

God's principle of process and preparation cannot be circumvented. Through the rough paths, God humbled and taught me the beauty of trusting Him to direct my life.

Thanks be to God Almighty Who in His infinite wisdom did not bestow such ability on me. I have realised that there is a purpose for the path God chose for me to walk in. God's principle of process and preparation cannot be circumvented. Through the rough paths, God humbled and taught me the beauty of trusting Him to direct my life (James 4:10). I was tried, processed and refined in the crucible of afflictions and adversity, until the fine qualities of my character were revealed. It was there in the crucible, that I developed the muscles of endurance and perseverance.

God is not haphazard in His doings. He is deliberate, precise and detailed in His planning and in His execution of His plans and purposes. He is the mighty God who rules in the affairs of men. He has been ruling the affairs of my life since the day I was conceived in my mother's womb.

I know that I am chosen in Christ Jesus and made God's heritage according to God's plan and in conformity with His purpose. I am not an afterthought. I am not an accident. I am a carefully crafted narrative in the detailed script of God's determined story. God has not and will not leave even the minute detail of my life to chance, coincidence or accident. He chose me in advance for this purpose that I, who put my trust and hope in God, will bring glory and praise to His name.

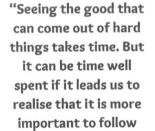

"Seeing the good that can come out of hard things takes time. But it can be time well spent if it leads us to realise that it is more important to follow God than to follow what we think is the best path for our lives."

I found that the script God crafted was His way of preparing me for my calling and mission. The humbling process turned out to be an opportunity to mature and develop as I pressed forward to apprehend the purpose for which God apprehended me.

The words of Lisa TerKeurst make a lot of sense to me now;

"Seeing the good that can come out of hard things takes time. But it can be time well spent if it leads us to realise that it is more important to follow God than to follow what we think is the best path for our lives."

I see each passing day the good God has purposed to bring out of my furnace experience. The time that it has taken for God's purpose to be made manifest has been time well spent. It is during this time of watching God's script unfold like a movie in the cinema that I found my calling. It was there that I discovered what God has called me to do in His Kingdom agenda.

God is connecting the dots. He is fixing each piece of the puzzle together. The picture is beginning to emerge. It is a beautiful picture. Each event in my story is a small piece of the amazing picture God has in mind for my future, standing alone they may be unclear and confusing but fitted together by the fingers of the Master Craftsman, the story of amazing grace begins to unfold.

> **My life story may have several chapters of misery, pain, and distress, but it is not a tragedy.**

My life story may have several chapters of misery, pain, and distress, but it is not a tragedy. I knew if I do not channel my season of pain and adversity to bring about good in the lives of others, then it would be in vain—indeed purposeless. If my story can become a means of inspiring hope and pointing others going through adversity to the Supreme Source of hope, then it would not be a story of tragedy but a story of victory.

That is the story you are holding in your hands today; the story of the grace of God that sustains through every valley of the shadow of death, through fiery furnace of affliction and through every adversity known to man. That grace is abundantly available to you come what may, wherever you may be and whatever you may be going through. God who kept me is still the same today. He is ready and waiting for you to turn to Him and put your trust in Him. He will do for you what He has done and is still doing for me—keep you and me by the power of His might hands and by His grace.

You can trust Him to connect the disjointed dots in your life. You can trust Him to put together the pieces of the puzzles lying in confusing disarray. He will do it if you only give it to Him. I believe that our season of affliction and adversity can become a unique opportunity to reach out and touch the lives of people in our community for good. I believe there's someone waiting at the end of our dark tunnel who can derive comfort from our experience if we refuse to give up on hope, if we refuse to give in to despair but push through to the end. I am persuaded that our story of pain and affliction can become a source of encouragement to others if we tap into the grace that is abundantly available to us.

Look out for **Beyond The Storms** – an unfolding of what God has called me to do and what God is using this story to accomplish in the lives of many people across the world.

Before you put this book down, I want you to pause and ponder on your relationship with God and with His Son, Jesus Christ. Have you accepted Jesus Christ as your Lord and Saviour? "For God so loved the world that He gave us His only begotten Son, that whosoever believes in Him should not perish but have everlasting life." It is only in Jesus Christ and through Him that you can connect with the grace that I have described in the book. This vital connection is established when you confess your sins and you accept Jesus Christ as your Lord and Saviour. If you made this decision to commit your life to Jesus Christ as your Lord today, please do not hesitate to contact us and to visit a Bible-believing church close to you.

May God's grace, blessings and peace continue to abound to you in increasing measures as you grow in your knowledge of Him.

DECLARATION

———■———

I know that I am chosen in Christ Jesus and made God's heritage according to God's plan and in conformity with His purpose. I am not an afterthought. I am not an accident. I am a carefully crafted narrative in the detailed script of God's determined story. God has not and will not leave even the minute detail of my life to chance, coincidence or accident. He chose me in advance for this purpose that I, who put my trust and hope in God, will bring glory and praise to His name.